# ACSM's
# HEALTH-RELATED
# PHYSICAL FITNESS
# ASSESSMENT MANUAL

## EDITORS

**GREGORY B. DWYER, PHD, FACSM**
Department of Movement Studies and Exercise Science
East Stroudsburg University of Pennsylvania
East Stroudsburg, Pennsylvania
and
**SHALA E. DAVIS, PHD, FACSM**
Department of Movement Studies and Exercise Science
East Stroudsburg University of Pennsylvania
East Stroudsburg, Pennsylvania

# ACSM's
# HEALTH-RELATED
# PHYSICAL FITNESS
# ASSESSMENT MANUAL

## AMERICAN COLLEGE OF SPORTS MEDICINE

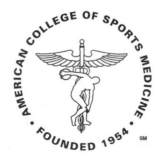

LIPPINCOTT WILLIAMS & WILKINS
A **Wolters Kluwer** Company
Philadelphia • Baltimore • New York • London
Buenos Aires • Hong Kong • Sydney • Tokyo

*Acquisitions Editor:* Peter J. Darcy
*Managing Editor:* Linda S. Napora
*Marketing Manager:* Christen DeMarco
*Production Editor:* Jennifer W. Glazer
*Designer:* Doug Smock
*Compositor:* LWW
*Printer:* Quebecor World—Dubuque

**Library of Congress Cataloging-in-Publication Data**

American College of Sports Medicine
    ACSM's health-related physical fitness assessment manual / editors, Gregory B. Dwyer and Shala E. Davis
        p. ; cm.
    Companion v. to ACSM's guidelines for exercise testing and prescription / American College of Sports Medicine ... [et al.]. 6th edition. c2000.
    Includes biographical references and index.
        ISBN 0-7817-3471-1
    1. Physical fitness—Testing. 2.2 Exercise tests. I. Title: Health-related physical fitness assessment manual. II. Dwyer, Gregory Byron 1959- III. Davis, Shala E. IV, American College of Sports Medicine. V. American College of Sports Medicine. ACSM's guidelines for exercise testing and prescription.
    [DNLM: 1. Physical Fitness. 2. Exercise Test—standards. 3. Physical Endurance. 4. Physical Examination—standards.]

GV436.A35 2004
613.7—dc22                                                                 2003060617

*The publishers have made every effort to trace the copyright holders for borrowed material. If they have inadvertently overlooked any, they will be pleased to make the necessary arrangements at the first opportunity.*

To purchase additional copies of this book, call our customer service department at **(800) 638-3030** or fax orders to **(301) 824-7390**. International customers should call **(301) 714-2324.**

***Visit Lippincott Williams & Wilkins on the Internet: http://www.LWW.com.*** Lippincott Williams & Wilkins customer service representatives are available from 8:30 am to 6:00 pm, EST.

06 07 08
4 5 6 7 8 9 10

# Preface

The goal of *ACSM's Health-Related Physical Fitness Assessment Manual* is to provide readers with the theory for developing skills in assessing health-related physical fitness and to offer guidelines for standard, step-by-step assessment procedures.

Chapters include an introduction and tests for each component of health-related physical fitness. The presentation of each assessment test covers standardized guidelines for collecting data on that given component as well as the normative guidelines or standards that can be used to interpret the results.

A unique feature of this manual is the step-by-step instructions (procedures) for each assessment so that the reader can easily learn the skills needed to collect the data and then practice those skills to become proficient. In addition, there are helpful laboratory exercises to be performed with some of the assessment tests, providing readers another opportunity for increasing proficiency. This manual contains numerous graphics (e.g., correct skinfolds anatomical sites), tables containing step-by-step instructions for each test, case studies that illustrate integration of all test data, and suggested readings that will direct the reader to additional information.

*ACSM's Health-Related Physical Fitness Assessment Manual* systematically unifies a field of study by presenting a single source to replace countless sources of this information (such as physical fitness texts, product information sources, measurement articles and texts). This manual closely follows the most current edition of *ACSM Guidelines for Exercise Testing and Prescription (GETP)*. There are numerous references to *ACSM's GETP* throughout the manual and thus the reader will need to have *ACSM's GETP* as a companion text. This manual is also designed to follow the ACSM certification level of Health/Fitness Instructor$_{SM}$ in terms of health-related physical fitness assessment.

This text covers the assessment of all five of the health-related components of physical fitness: (1) cardiorespiratory fitness, (2) body composition, (3) muscular strength, (4) muscular endurance, and (5) flexibility. Features include:

- The subject area presented in this manual is covered in its entirety and with depth; more so than in any other reference.
- Assessment tests presented in a cookbook recipe format to help the user perform the assessment on a client.
- Chapters follow the knowledge, skills, and abilities (KSAs) necessary for the ACSM certification of Health/Fitness Instructor$_{SM}$ in the area of health-related physical fitness assessment.
- Pre-Activity Screening and ACSM Risk Stratification and the definitions of Physical Fitness.
- More than 50 physical fitness assessment tests are covered in step-by-step procedures, along with normative data to assist in interpreting results.
- Practice problems, case studies, and laboratory exercises provide additional learning opportunities.

We have all come to appreciate the wisdom that "keeping fit" is the key to a healthier and longer life. If this manual makes a contribution to that goal, our purpose in writing this text will be fulfilled.

# Credits

The authors gratefully acknowledge the following publishers who granted permission for reproduction of illustrations and tables as noted:

**American College of Sports Medicine. ACSM's Guidelines for Exercise Testing and Prescription, 6th ed. Philadelphia: Lippincott Williams & Wilkins, 2000.**
Box 1-2 (pgs 5 6), Box 2-1 (pg 26), Box 2-2 (pg 24), Box 2-3 (pg 25), Table 2-1 (pg 27), Figure 3-3 (pg 118), Table 3-1 (pg 41), Table 3-2 (pg 119), Table 4-3 (pg 64), Table 4-6 (pg 62), Box 4-1 (pg 65), Box 4-2 (pg 66), Table 5-2 (pg 82), Table 5-3 (pg 83), Table 5-4 (pg 86), Table 5-5 (pg 85), Table 5-7 (pg 88), Table 5-8 (pg 88), Box 5-1 (pg 84), Box 5-2 (pg 87), Table 6-1 (pg 77), Figure 7-2 (pg 75), Figure 7-3 (pg 76), Figure 7-4 (pg 73), Box 7-2 (pg 80), Box 7-3 (pg 72), Box 7-5 (pg 74), Figure 8-1 (pg 98), Box 8-1 (pg 102), Box 8-2 (pg 50), Box 8-3 (pg 104)

**American College of Sports Medicine. ACSM's Resource Manual for Guidelines for Exercise Testing and Prescription, 4th ed. Philadelphia: Lippincott Williams & Wilkins, 2001.**
Figure 3-2 (pg 97), Figure 3-4 (pg 98), Figure 3-5 (pg 98), Figure 4-2 (pg 103), Figure 4-3 (pg 102), Figure 4-4 (pg 102), Figure 4-5 (pg 101), Figure 4-6 (pg 102), Figure 4-7 (pg 102), Figure 4-8 (pg 99), Table 4-2 (pg 393), Table 4-4 (pg 394)

**Bray GA. Obesity: definition, diagnosis and disadvantages. Med J Australia 1985;142:S2-S8.**
Figure 4-1

**Brown SP. Introduction to Exercise Science. Baltimore: Lippincott Williams & Wilkins, 2001.**
Figure 7-1 (pg 219)

**Canadian Physical Activity, Fitness & Lifestyle Appraisal, 2nd ed. 1998 (with permission from the Canadian Society for Exercise Physiology).**
Table 5-1 (pg 641)

**Golding LA, ed. YMCA Fitness Testing and Assessment Manual, 4th ed. 2000 (with permission of the YMCA of the USA, 101 North Wacker Drive, Chicago, IL 60606).**
Table 5-6 (pg 200-211)

**Kaminsky LA, Whaley MW. Evaluation of a new standardized ramp protocol: the BSU/Bruce Ramp Protocol. J Cardiopulm Rehabil 1998;18:438 444.**
Table 8-4 (pgs 438-444)

**McCardle WD, Katch FI, Katch VL. Essentials of Exercise Physiology. Philadelphia, Lippincott Williams & Wilkins, 2000.**
Table 4-1 (pg 502), Table 4-5 (pgs 654-660)

# Acknowledgments

We thank all who generously contributed their time and expertise in bringing this book to fruition: our reviewers at the American College of Sports Medicine—especially Lenny Kaminsky, Mark Kasper, Jeff Roitman, and Mitch Whaley; our colleagues and students at East Stroudsburg University of Pennsylvania and around the country; and our editorial, marketing, and production team at Lippincott Williams & Wilkins—especially Pete Darcy, Linda Napora, Christen DeMarco, and Jenn Weir Glazer.

Most of all, we thank our spouses and children for their love and encouragement—Beth Dwyer and my sons, Kevin and Eric Dwyer, and John Kochmansky and my son, Jake Kochmansky. We are so fortunate that there are so many people who are always there for us.

—*G.B.D.* and *S.E.D.*

# Contents

# 1

# Introduction

## DEFINING PHYSICAL FITNESS

Physical fitness assessment is the focus of this manual. Physical fitness is a dynamic construct in that it is continually growing in importance to everyday life and health. If you are going to measure or assess the construct of physical fitness, then you need to know the definition of *physical fitness*. Unfortunately there are many definitions of this construct. The President's Council on Physical Fitness and Sport has composed an often-cited definition of physical fitness.

> *"Physical fitness is the ability to carry out daily tasks with vigor and alertness without undue fatigue and ample energy to enjoy leisure time pursuits and meet unforeseen emergencies." (President's Council on Physical Fitness and Sport)*

However, the above definition of physical fitness from the President's Council can be criticized for its lack of objectivity in measurement. When the objectivity of a definition can be questioned then it may be difficult to measure or assess that term. Specifically, the use of terms "vigor" and "alertness" along with "undue fatigue" and "ample energy" causes this definition of physical fitness to be subjective and to defy measurement. Since terms in the definition of physical fitness also need defining, it is difficult to devise specific measurement tools to measure or assess physical fitness.

One of the founders in the field of physical fitness is Leroy 'Bud' Getchell, PhD, professor emeritus of Ball State University. Dr. Getchell defined physical fitness in one of his textbooks.

> *"Physical fitness is the capability of the heart, blood vessels, lungs and muscles to perform at optimal efficiency." (Bud Getchell, PhD)*

While this may be a 'fine' definition of the construct of physical fitness, it lacks the ability for simple measurement. There are several other definitions for physical fitness. Below is a selection of some of these many definitions:

> *"Physical fitness is the ability to perform moderate to vigorous levels of physical activity without undue fatigue and the capability of maintaining such ability throughout life." (American College of Sports Medicine)*

> *"Physical fitness is a set of attributes that people have or achieve that relates to the ability to perform physical activity." (U.S. Centers for Disease Control and Prevention)*

Indeed there have been numerous definitions of physical fitness as is pointed out in the next statement:

> *"Physical fitness is one of the most poorly defined and most frequently misused terms in the English Language." (Brian Sharkey, PhD, professor emeritus of University of Montana)*

'Poor' definitions that have vague, subjective wording and definitions made up of terms that also need defining have led to the confusion over what is physical fitness. Thus, many of the definitions of physical fitness lack the ability to lead the fitness professional towards a way of measuring physical fitness until one considers the definitions of Health-Related physical fitness below.

| BOX 1-1 | A Comparison Between the Health-Related and Athletic Ability Components of Physical Fitness. |
|---------|---------------------------------------------------------------------------------------------------|

| Health-Related Components | Athletic Ability Components (Performance or Skill-Related *(not inclusive)* |
|---------------------------|----------------------------------------------------------------------------|
| Cardiorespiratory Fitness | Balance |
| Body Composition | Reaction Time |
| Flexibility | Coordination |
| Muscular Strength | Agility |
| Muscular Endurance | Speed |
| | Power |

## HEALTH-RELATED PHYSICAL FITNESS

*"The five health-related components of physical fitness are more important to public health than are the components related to athletic ability. Operational definitions of physical fitness vary with the interest and need of the investigators." (U.S. Centers for Disease Control and Prevention)*

The definition of physical fitness offered by the U.S. Centers for Disease Control and Prevention focuses on the difference between health-related physical fitness and athletic ability physical fitness. From the perspective of the health of the nation, often referred to as the public health perspective, the health-related components are more important than those related to athletic ability (or are skill-related or performance-related components.) The distinction between the health-related versus the athletic ability components of physical fitness is shown in Box 1-1.

Thus, health-related physical fitness assessment can be, and should be, divided into the components that make up the whole construct. All five of the health-related components contribute equally, or are in balance, to the whole of health-related physical fitness (see Fig. 1-1). The approach of dividing up health-related physical fitness into the components that make up the whole construct allows for its measurement.

**HEALTH-RELATED PHYSICAL FITNESS
A BALANCE BETWEEN THE COMPONENTS**

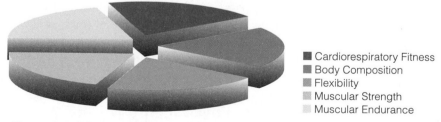

■ Cardiorespiratory Fitness
■ Body Composition
■ Flexibility
■ Muscular Strength
■ Muscular Endurance

**FIGURE 1-1.** A balance between all five of the components of health-related physical fitness.

## Components of Health-Related Physical Fitness

Cardiorespiratory fitness is related to the ability to perform large muscle, dynamic, moderate-to-high intensity exercise for prolonged periods. Cardiorespiratory fitness can be assessed by various techniques and has many synonyms. One such synonym is maximal aerobic capacity (see Chapters 6 through 8).

Body composition refers to the relative percentage of body weight that is fat and fat-free tissue. Percent body fat, among other techniques, may be used to assess body composition (see Chapter 4 ).

Flexibility is the ability to move a joint through its complete range of movement. Flexibility depends on which muscle and joint are being evaluated; therefore, it is joint-specific (see Chapter 5).

Muscular strength refers to the maximal force that can be generated by a specific muscle or muscle group (see Chapter 5). Muscular endurance is the ability of a muscle group to execute repeated contractions over time sufficient enough to cause muscular fatigue, or to maintain a specific percentage of the maximum voluntary contraction for a prolonged period of time (see Chapter 5). Muscular strength and muscular endurance can be combined into one component of health-related physical fitness titled *muscular fitness*; this term has been used to describe the integrated status of muscular strength and muscular endurance.

## Total Physical Fitness

An interesting question that could be asked is: if the definition of physical fitness includes or is made up of five health-related components, then how does one measure or express the concept of total physical fitness?

If you ponder this question for a while, you may note the futility of the notion of measuring or expressing total physical fitness. Thus, the concept of total physical fitness is abandoned for a component model (cardiorespiratory fitness or body composition). The measurement of physical fitness also is broken down into measuring each of the five health-related components separately. Each individual component of health-related physical fitness is then compared to the appropriate normative (norms) data for the individual. There is then no attempt in this manual to figure some composite score for total physical fitness.

## Tests for Components of Health-Related Physical Fitness

The approach to measuring health-related physical fitness is to measure, or assess, each component of the whole construct separately. A test is defined as a static instrument or tool that is used to measure or assess. There are several tests that purport to measure any given component of health-related physical fitness. Evaluation is a dynamic process designed around deciding on your client's specific health-related physical fitness. These tests vary in their complexity, validity, reliability, and measurement costs, as is explored later in this manual. Figure 1-2 presents examples of some of the tests that measure or assess individual components of health-related physical fitness (these tests are discussed in this manual).

## Importance of Health-Related Physical Fitness

Many adults can be and should be both more physically active and more physically fit. Many reports, both laboratory-based and epidemiological, show the need for this more

| Cardiorespiratory Fitness: | Body Composition: | Muscular Strength: |
|---|---|---|
| • Field Tests: i.e., Step Tests, 1.5 Mile Walk/Run, One Mile Walk Test | • Height/Weight & Body Mass Index | • Hand Grip Test |
| | • Circumferences & Waist-to-Hip Ratio | • One RM (repetition maximum) |
| • Submaximal Tests: i.e., YMCA Submaximal Cycle Test & Astrand-Ryhming Cycle Test | • Skinfolds | Muscular Endurance: |
| | • Bioelectrical Impedance | • Sit-ups |
| | • Underwater Weighing | • Curl-ups |
| | Flexibility: | • Pushups |
| • Maximal Tests: Graded Exercise Test | • Sit and Reach Test | • YMCA Bench Press Test |
| | • Modified Sit and Reach Test | |

FIGURE 1-2. A sampling of the tests that may be used to measure each individual component of health-related physical fitness. *Note: Muscular strength and muscular endurance can be combined into one component of health-related physical fitness titled muscular fitness. There are more individual test items for each component of health-related physical fitness than can displayed in this figure.* In addition, there are some other test items, such as resting metabolic rate, that are covered in this manual that do not fit easily into this figure.

physically active lifestyle. This is expressed well in the 1996 report from the U.S. Surgeon General (*Physical Activity and Health; A Report of the Surgeon General*); however, one national survey reported that approximately 12% of adult Americans (over the age of 18 years) are regularly physically active in vigorous exercise. Thus, as fitness professionals, an important task we all have is to get more Americans active.

Because of the alarming statistics on the lack of physical fitness and activity in the U.S. (and in the world) adult population, along with the strong evidence for the many benefits of physical activity on health, several national reports and campaigns have been issued in an attempt to increase physical activity. The recent U.S. Surgeon General report thoroughly examined the importance of physical activity and also stressed the importance of a pre-activity screening (see Chapter 2). Also inherent in this need to increase activity among all Americans is the need to perform selected physical fitness assessments on potential clients. Some of the many benefits of being physically active are listed in Box 1-2.

## Measuring Health-Related Physical Fitness

The measurement or assessment of health-related physical fitness is a fairly common practice by fitness professionals. Several reasons to measure each component of health-related physical fitness are to:

• Educate individuals about their current health-related physical fitness
• Use data from the assessments to individualize exercise programs
• Provide baseline and follow-up data to evaluate exercise programs
• Motivate individuals towards more specific action/exercise
• Help with client's risk stratification

Each client and situation is different, thus, the reason for performing a health-related physical fitness assessment for each client may vary.

| BOX 1-2 | Benefits of Regular Physical Activity and/or Exercise* |

*Improvement in Cardiovascular and Respiratory Function*
- Increased maximal oxygen uptake due to both central and peripheral adaptations
- Lower minute ventilation at a given submaximal intensity
- Lower myocardial oxygen cost for a given absolute submaximal intensity
- Lower heart rate and blood pressure at a given submaximal intensity
- Increased capillary density in skeletal muscle
- Increased exercise threshold for the accumulation of lactate in the blood
- Increased exercise threshold for the onset of disease signs or symptoms (e.g., angina pectoris, ischemic ST-segment depression, claudication)

*Reduction in Coronary Artery Disease Risk Factors*
- Reduced resting systolic/diastolic pressures
- Increased serum high-density lipoprotein cholesterol and decreased serum triglycerides
- Reduced total body fat, reduced intra-abdominal fat
- Reduced insulin needs, improved glucose tolerance

*Decreased Mortality and Morbidity*
Primary prevention (i.e., interventions to prevent an acute cardiac event)
1. activity and/or fitness levels are associated with lower death rates from coronary artery disease
2. Higher activity and/or fitness levels are associated with lower incidence rates for combined cardiovascular diseases, coronary artery disease, cancer of the colon, and type 2 diabetes
   - Secondary prevention (i.e., interventions after a cardiac event [to prevent another])
3. Based on meta-analyses (pooled data across studies), cardiovascular and all-cause mortality are reduced in post-myocardial infarction patients who participate in cardiac rehabilitation exercise training, especially as a component of multifactorial risk factor reduction
4. Randomized controlled trials of cardiac rehabilitation exercise training involving post-myocardial infarction patients do not support a reduction in the rate of nonfatal reinfarction

*Other Postulated Benefits*
- Decreased anxiety and depression
- Enhanced feelings of well-being
- Enhanced performance of work, recreational, and sport activities

*Adapted from United States Department of Health and Human Services. Physical activity and health: a report of the Surgeon General. Atlanta, GA: US Department of Health and Human Services, Centers for Disease Control and Prevention, National Center for Chronic Disease Prevention and Health Promotion, 1996; Pollock ML, Gaesser GA, Butcher JD. The recommended quantity and quality of exercise for developing and maintaining cardiorespiratory and muscular fitness, and flexibility in healthy adults. Med Sci Sports Exerc 1998;30:975-991; Franklin BA, Roitman JL. Cardiorespiratory adaptations to exercise. In: Roitman JL, ed. ACSM's Resource Manual for Guidelines for Exercise Testing and Prescription. Baltimore: Williams & Wilkins, 1998:156-163; Wenger NK, Froelicher ES, Smith LK, et al. Cardiac rehabilitation. Clinical practice guidelines No. 17. Rockville, MD: US Department of Health and Human Services, Public Health Service, Agency for Health Care Policy and Research and the National Heart, Lung and Blood Institute, AHCPR Publication No. 96-0672, October 1995; and Whaley MH, Kaminsky LA. Epidemiology of physical activity, physical fitness and selected chronic diseases. In: Roitman JL, ed. ACSM's Resource Manual for Guidelines for Exercise Testing and Prescription. Baltimore: Williams & Wilkins, 1998:13-26.

## Health-Related Physical Fitness, Exercise, and Physical Activity

Because of the public's perception or misperception about health-related physical fitness and physical activity and exercise there is a need to define these terms. Unfortunately, the scientific literature and lay public often use the terms incorrectly or interchangeably. This can result in misunderstandings. This manual has previously defined health-related physical fitness in a component model as a set of attributes an individual has or possesses, such as cardiorespiratory fitness or flexibility.

Exercise represents structured, planned activities designed to promote or enhance overall physical fitness, not just health-related physical fitness. Examples of exercises include swimming or jogging.

Physical activity is any bodily movement, regardless of intensity, that is not designed specifically around the purpose of enhancing physical fitness. Some examples of physical activity are walking your pet or taking a shower; however, certain forms or intensities of Physical Activity (such as walking your pet) may be beneficial to overall health and wellness. Thus, the fitness professional must ensure that the public does not confuse health-related physical fitness with physical activity or exercise.

## TESTING AND MEASUREMENT PRIMER

There are several tests for each of the five components of health-related physical fitness. The choice of which specific test to use for any individual component can be difficult. Some items to consider in making a choice include:

- Ease of test administration
- Ease of normative data comparison
- Other economy issues, such as the cost of a given test
- Validity and accuracy of test results

When choosing the particular test best suited for a client and environment, the ease of test administration is one important factor. Ease of test administration means just that: how easy is it to have a client perform that given test? Included in ease of test administration is the issue of how easy is it for the fitness professional and the client to interact in performing the test. Some tests, such as the skinfold procedure for body composition, are relatively easy to administer; others, such as underwater weighing for body composition, are more difficult. It may make sense to choose a particular test that is easier to administer to certain clients based on the testing conditions. It should become more apparent which of these tests is easier to administer and interpret than others as the test procedures are presented in each chapter.

A separate factor to consider is just how applicable and well developed the normative standards (norms) are for a given test. There are several questions that should be considered by all fitness professionals in this area:

- Can a client's achievement on a particular test be compared to a similar group of subjects?
- Who or for what group are the norms for that particular test based on?
- Are the norms criterion-referenced standards or are they normative standards?

There is further information on criterion-referenced standards versus normative standards later in this chapter. After the administration of a particular test to a client, the issue of just how applicable are the standards or norms used to interpret the test results becomes important.

Some of the assessments that are more commonly used for health-related physical fitness have more thoroughly developed standards than do other assessments. A discussion of each of the health-related physical fitness assessments and their interpretation can be found in their respective chapters.

There are also other economy issues on which to base the selection of which test to use, such as budget costs (i.e., equipment costs), staff and training needs, and the ability of clients to understand the test procedures and results. With the discussion of each particular health-related physical fitness assessment test, there will be mention of the equipment needs for that particular assessment.

Finally, the validity of test results versus the need for accuracy in test results should be considered. Validity and accuracy are discussed further in the next section of this manual. A word of caution is offered: there are no perfect tests in the area of health-related physical fitness. The fitness professional will have to make some decisions on which test to use and undoubtedly will have to make some compromises in that decision.

## Test Choice Considerations

With the use of a particular test, there is the need to answer several questions related to sound testing and measurement practice:

1. How can one be sure that the test item measures what it is designed to measure?

   The ability of a test to measure specifically what it is designed to measure is known as the validity of the test. For example, the measurement of skinfold thicknesses at selected anatomical sites has been suggested as a valid assessment of percent body fat for body composition evaluation. The validity of skinfold thickness assessment to estimate body density and body composition will be discussed further in Chapter 4. The validity of a test item is generally demonstrated by comparing the test item measure to some 'gold standard' assessment for that particular component. In the case of skinfolds, researchers have compared skinfold measurement to underwater weighing (the often-considered gold standard for percent body fat) to demonstrate the validity of skinfold measurement for percent body fat or body composition. In other words, validity refers to the ability of a test to measure a particular item.

   Validity may be expressed several ways: two such ways are as a correlation coefficient (r) or as a standard error of the estimate (SEE). Both the correlation coefficient and the standard error of the estimate will be discussed later in this chapter. The validity of a particular test is considered by some to be the most important consideration in test choice. There are several sub-components of validity that will not be discussed here such as content validity and construct validity.

   Also, the term accuracy, which is a measure of how exacting or correct a test score is, can be considered similar to the validity of a test. Accuracy may be easily thought of in terms of how subjective or objective is the scoring method for a test. Accuracy can also be ascribed to a piece of equipment used in testing procedure. A simple way of summing up the term accuracy is "is the score correct?"

2. Would the individual get the same score if they were tested a second time?

   This is known as the reliability of the test item. Another way of phrasing reliability is: "Is there consistency or repeatability of a test score across different testing conditions?" One test measurement procedure is to have a subject perform multiple trials of a test and then use the best score as the measure for comparison purposes; this score is taken partially because of the reliability of that particular test item. One way to measure the reliability of a test using the test-retest method is with a correlation coefficient (r). The correlation coefficient for test-retest reliability is simply a comparison between two scores for a particular test for a particular individual, or how similar are the set of scores for a particular individual.

## Pretest Instructions, Environment, and Order

By paying attention to the details of the testing session, it is proposed that the validity and reliability of a client's test results can be increased, which will give a more accurate picture of the health-related physical fitness. Details of the testing session include any pretest instructions given to an individual, the physical surroundings or environment of the testing session, and the order of the tests if multiple tests are going to be performed in one testing session. In the *Guidelines for Exercise Testing and Prescription (GETP)* from the American College of Sports Medicine, these issues are discussed and summary tables are provided. Thus, the reader of this manual is referred to the most current edition of the *GETP* for further information. A summary of the information contained in *GETP* is provided in the following section.

General Pretest Instructions:
- wear loose-fitting, comfortable clothes that will easily allow a person to perform a particular test
- avoid food, alcohol, and caffeine for at least 3 hours before the test
- drink plenty of fluids during the preceding 24 hours until the test
- avoid strenuous exercise on the day of the test
- get plenty of rest or sleep (6–8 hours) on the night before the test

General Test Environment:
- the room temperature should be between 70° and 74°F (21°–23°C)
- the room should be quiet and private
- the room should be well ventilated

General Test Order:
- have all paperwork and forms ready before the test
- organize and calibrate all equipment ahead of time
- the test session should not be rushed for time
- there should be clear explanation of all procedures
- perform all resting measures first; then evaluate cardiorespiratory fitness assessments before doing tests of muscular fitness

## Testing Session Organization: Resting Versus Exercise Testing

Using specific tests and measures, one can assess all health-related physical fitness components. These tests and measures may be divided into two groups by the activity that a particular test item requires of the client or subject (Box 1-3). For example, one group of tests may be categorized as resting (or quiet) tests because the tests employed require little exertion on the part of the participant. In fact, resting or quiet tests generally demand that the subject be relaxed and free of stimulants at the time of testing for more accurate results. The second group of tests falls under the category of exercise tests. Exercise tests require some exertion by the participant to complete the test. The mix of testing employed may dictate the testing session. For instance, if resting measurements are to be taken, they may have to be done on a separate day from when exercise tests are to be performed.

| BOX 1-3 | The Division Between Resting and Exercise Tests |
|---------|-------------------------------------------------|

| Resting (Quiet) tests include: | Exercise tests include: |
|--------------------------------|-------------------------|
| Resting Blood Pressure and Heart Rate | Flexibility Tests |
| Body Composition | Muscular Strength Tests |
| | Muscular Endurance Tests |
| | Field Tests for Prediction of Cardiorespiratory Fitness |
| | Submaximal Tests for Prediction of Cardiorespiratory Fitness |
| | Maximal Graded Exercise Tests |

## Test Score Interpretation: Criterion-Referenced Standards Versus Normative Data

Once a test has been performed on a client, the test results should be interpreted. The interpretation of these results traditionally depends on the use of some comparison to a set of standards or norms. There are basically two types of standards: criterion-referenced standards and normative standards. Criterion-referenced standards are a set of scores that would be 'desirable' to achieve based on external criteria such as the betterment of health (a group of 'experts' may have to agree on what a 'desirable' score may be for that particular test). While criterion-referenced standards may be thought of as desirable, they are open to subjective interpretation and open to criticism. Criterion-referenced standards may thus use adjectives such as 'excellent' or 'poor' in the data interpretation tables. Normative standards, sometimes shortened to norms, are based on the past performance of a group of like or similar individuals. With norms, a comparison is made between how the client performed and how other, similar individuals faired. The data interpretation tables may then use a percentile score, such as '90th ' or '50th' , etc. Evaluative decisions about a client's health-related physical fitness can be based on either criterion-referenced standards or normative standards. In the health-related physical fitness assessment arena, more individual tests have normative standards associated with them than have criterion-referenced standards. Criterion-referenced standards exist mostly in the cardiorespiratory fitness ($\dot{V}O_{2max}$) and body composition (percent body fat) areas. Even though criterion-referenced norms may exist in these areas, there is still disagreement among 'experts' as to what they mean. Some of the questions to consider regarding the use of standards are:

- Are the norms for a test specific to different ages and genders?
- Do the norms represent the entire population for scores, from low to high?
- How do you interpret norms that use descriptors such as 'excellent,' 'average,' 'poor'? Are these descriptors fair?

There is a growing trend in the assessment of health-related physical fitness towards not using any set of standards when evaluating a client's raw score. The client's raw score may only be used to compare to future or past results of that client for that same test. Thus, there is less concern about whether the norms for a particular test are 'appropriate' for that client; in essence, clients are compared only to themselves over time (such as over the course of an exercise training program).

## Prediction Error and Testing

Many health-related physical fitness tests predict a score for the component being measured. Some examples of this prediction are skinfold thickness for body composition and the submaximal cycle ergometer test for cardiorespiratory fitness. While the individual test (i.e., skinfolds) is a measure of that component of health-related physical fitness (i.e., body composition), there is a prediction made from the skinfold thickness test score to the percentage of body fat (body composition). Since prediction is an important part of health-related physical fitness testing, it is worth some explanation.

First, if you are going to predict, then you must accept that there is going to be some error in that prediction. The measurement error in the prediction of a test score can be expressed as the standard error of the estimate (SEE) presented previously in the validity section. This SEE refers to the bell-shaped curve and the normal distribution of scores in the population. Similar to the Standard Deviation (SD), the SEE is generally expressed as a ± of the score. One SEE unit refers to 67% of the population; or 67% of the population will be within the score ± the SEE. Thus, the SEE can be used to express the validity of a particular test item. An example of the use of the SEE in health-related physical fitness assessment is found below.

The correlation coefficient may also be reported for a specific test item. The correlation coefficient, expressed as the small letter r, is a mathematical expression of the relationship between items or variables. The correlation coefficient is used to express the relationship between a test item score that is predicted versus an actual measurement of the same, or different, test item. This relationship can be positive ($r \approx +0.X$), negative ($r \approx -0.X$), or close to zero ($r \approx 0.0$). A positive relationship means that as one test item score increases so does the other test item. A negative relationship means as one score increases, the other decreases. The r is useful to establish whether a test item is measuring what it is designed to measure (validity), and if a test score can be repeated (test-retest reliability). There is an example of the correlation coefficient in health-related physical fitness assessment found below.

## Standard Error of Estimate

The age-prediction of maximal heart rate (HRmax), in beats per minute (bpm), can be predicted from the following equation: HRmax = 220 − age (years). This mathematical formula has a SEE associated with it of about SEE = ± 12 bpm. Thus, a 22-year-old client would have an age-predicted HRmax of (220 − 22 = 198 bpm) of 198 beats per minute. However, the SEE is ± 12 bpm, thus, 67% (or two-thirds) of all 22-year-old clients may have a HRmax between 186 and 210 bpm (198 ± 12 bpm) when measured at maximal exercise in the lab on a treadmill. Using this prediction formula, 33% (or one-third) of all 22-year-old clients will have a measured HRmax greater than 210 bpm or less than 186 bpm. But, all 22-year-old clients who use the age-predicted HRmax formula will be told their age-predicted HRmax is 198 bpm by this prediction equation. This example of potential error is applicable to the prediction error of submaximal exercise testing.

The SEE for one of the Jackson and Pollock skinfold equations for percent body fat is SEE = ± 3.8%. This means that if you measure (and thus, predict) an individual's percent body fat by skinfold thickness using one of the Jackson and Pollock formulas there is ± 3.8% error in the measurement. Or, in practical terms, if you measure an individual's skinfolds and predict the body fat percentage to be 20%, then 67% of similar individuals (with the same sum of skinfolds) will be between 16.2% and 23.8% body fat as a range. Thirty-three percent will be even further away from the 20% (<

16.2 % or > 23.8%) predicted for them from the sum of their skinfolds. Further discussion of this topic appears in the Anthropometry and Body Composition chapter (Chapter 4).

## Correlations

The correlation coefficient between underwater weighing and the 7-site skinfold thickness formula by Jackson and Pollock for men for percent body fat is r = +0.88. This means that the relationship is positive (as one increases, so does the other) between these two tests—7-site skinfold thickness and the 'gold-standard' of underwater weighing. The correlation coefficient, however, is not 1.0, but less than 1.0 or 0.88. The relationship is not perfect. This would be one way of expressing the validity of skinfold thickness measurement by comparing it to the 'gold-standard' measurement of underwater weighing.

You can, however, reduce the error and increase the accuracy inherent in many health-related physical fitness assessments by:

- doing a good job of preparing your client for the testing session (i.e., avoiding stimulants ahead of time)
- organizing your testing session (i.e., calibrating all of your equipment)
- paying attention to the test details (i.e., achieving steady-state heart rates during the submaximal cycle ergometer tests)
- performing multiple trials (i.e., performing multiple skinfold thickness measures at one site for body composition analysis).

## SUMMARY

The assessment of health-related physical fitness is best accomplished by measuring each of the five individual components of health-related physical fitness. However, measuring these individual components is not an exact science. In fact, much of the assessment of health-related physical fitness depends on prediction techniques and is prone to error. Therefore, you should not 'over-interpret' the assessment results on your client, but rather use the assessment results as a tool to encourage greater commitment of your client to overall health-related physical fitness. Always remember, assessment should be an instrument to encourage increased physical activity and exercise and not be an end in itself.

### Suggested Readings

1. American College of Sports Medicine. ACSM's Guidelines for Exercise Testing and Prescription. 6th edition. Baltimore: Lippincott Williams & Wilkins, 2000.
2. Pate RR. The evolving definition of physical fitness. Quest 1988:40:174-179.
3. Physical Activity and Health: A Report of the Surgeon General. Atlanta, GA: US Department of Health and Human Services, Centers for Disease Control and Prevention, National Center for Chronic Disease Prevention and Health Promotion, 1996.
4. American College of Sports Medicine. ACSM's Resource Manual for Guidelines for Exercise Testing and Prescription. 4th edition. Baltimore: Lippincott Williams & Wilkins, 2001.
5. Whaley MH, Kaminsky LA. Epidemiology of physical activity, physical fitness and selected chronic diseases. In: ACSM's Resource Manual for Guidelines for Exercise Testing and Prescription. 4th edition. Baltimore: Lippincott Williams & Wilkins, 2001.

# 2

# Pre-Activity Screening

Pre-activity screening is the first step in the process of health-related physical fitness assessment. Pre-activity screening is a process of gathering a client's demographic and health-related information, along with some medical/health assessments, such as resting blood pressure, to aid decision-making on a client's health-related physical activity assessment and exercise future. The pre-activity screening is also a dynamic process in that it may vary in its scope and components depending on the client's needs from a medical/health standpoint (e.g., they have some form of disease), the type of health-related physical fitness assessments gathered (e.g., submaximal versus maximal cardiovascular endurance tests), and the physical activity program goals (e.g., moderate versus vigorous exercise).

Some of the reasons why clients should be screened for participation in health-related physical fitness assessment programs:

- To identify those with a medical contraindication (exclusion) to performing specific health-related physical fitness assessments.
- To identify those who should receive a medical/physician evaluation/examination before performing specific health-related physical fitness assessments.
- To identify those who should participate in a medically supervised health-related physical fitness assessment and/or program.
- To identify those with other health/medical concerns. (i.e., diabetes mellitus, orthopedic injuries, readiness for exercise, etc.)

## PRE-ACTIVITY SCREENING GUIDELINES

To reduce the occurrence of any unwanted event during a health-related physical fitness assessment or during an exercise program, it is prudent to conduct some form of pre-activity screening on a client. There are many national organizations, including the American College of Sports Medicine (ACSM), that have made suggestions as to just what these pre-activity screening guidelines should be; however, it is helpful to remember that these are just suggestions or guidelines.

In the 1996 report on Physical Activity and Health, the U.S. Surgeon General stated that:

> *"Previously inactive men over age 40, women over age 50, and people at high risk for CVD should first consult a physician before embarking on a program of vigorous physical activity to which they are unaccustomed. People with disease should be evaluated by a physician first..."*

In addition, a summary of the 'cautions' listed on many of the pieces of current exercise equipment, in exercise books, and on videos is:
"First consult your physician before starting an exercise program.
This is especially important for:
- Men ≥ 45 years old; Women ≥ 55 years old
- Those who are going to perform vigorous physical activity
- And for those who are new to exercise or are unaccustomed to exercise"

Per Olaf Åstrand, a famous Scandinavian exercise physiologist, once stated:

> *"Anyone who is in doubt about the condition of his health should consult his physician. But as a general rule, moderate activity is less harmful to health than inactivity."*

There are several components of the pre-activity screening, including:

- Medical History/Health Habits Questionnaire
- Physical Activity Readiness Questionnaire (PAR-Q)
- Medical/Health Exam

## Medical History/Health Habits Questionnaire

Some form of a Health History Questionnaire (HHQ) is necessary to use with a client to establish their medical/health risks for both exercise testing and participation in an exercise program. The HHQ, along with other medical/health data, is used in the process of risk stratification discussed later in this chapter. An example of a HHQ form is included in Appendix C as a sample. The HHQ should be tailored to fit the needs of the program as far as asking for the specific information needed from a client. In general, the HHQ should assess (among other things) a client's:

- Family history
- History of various diseases and illnesses including cardiovascular disease
- Surgical history
- Past and present health behaviors/habits (such as history of cigarette smoking and physical activity)
- Current use of various drugs/medications
- Specific history of various signs and symptoms suggesting cardiovascular disease among other things

The current edition of *ACSM's Guidelines for Exercise Testing and Prescription* (*GETP*) contains a more detailed list of the specifics of the medical history. Again, fitness professionals should tailor the HHQ to their own and their client's specific needs. In 1998 the American Heart Association and the ACSM put together a list of pre-participation screening guidelines for health and fitness programs that can be followed.

## Physical Activity Readiness Questionnaire (PAR-Q)

The HHQ is generally thought of as being a fairly comprehensive assessment of a client's medical and health history. Because the HHQ can be more information than is needed in some situations, the Physical Activity Readiness Questionnaire, or PAR-Q, was developed in Canada to be simpler in both scope and use. The PAR-Q is a form that contains seven YES-NO questions that have been found to be both readable and understandable for an individual to answer. The PAR-Q is designed to screen clients from participating in physical activities that may be too strenuous for them. The PAR-Q has been recommended as a minimal standard for entry into moderate intensity exercise programs. Thus, at the very least, a prudent fitness professional should consider having their clients fill out a PAR-Q, if appropriate. A copy of the PAR-Q is found in Appendix C of this manual.

## Medical/Health Examination

A medical examination led by a physician (or other qualified medical personnel) may also be necessary or desirable to help evaluate the health status of the client before further health-related physical fitness assessment. The suggested components of this medical examination can be found in the most current edition of the ACSM *GETP*. In addition to a medical examination, it may be desirable to perform some routine laboratory assessments on your client before performing more extensive health-related physical fitness assessment.

## RISK STRATIFICATION

The ACSM has a specific set of guidelines for pre-activity screening termed *risk stratification*.

To stratify is to divide or separate into levels or classes, called strata. The purpose of risk stratification is to help decide on the appropriate course of action regarding exercise testing when screening an individual before entering an exercise program. There are three 'risk stratification' classes or strata developed for individuals for this purpose (Box 2-1).

Specifically, the ACSM risk stratification guidelines suggest:

- Should a client have a medical examination (including a Graded Exercise Test [GXT]) before starting an exercise program?
- Does a client need a physician to be present for supervision of their GXT?

### ACSM Guidelines: Risk Stratification Strata

The three risk stratification strata or classes (low, moderate, and high risk) can be used to help decide on an appropriate course of action for a client regarding the need for a medical examination before any health-related physical fitness assessment. Always remember, however, that these are guidelines and one must also exercise clinical, prudent judgment as far as whether a client needs to see a physician first for clearance.

### ACSM Coronary Artery Disease Risk Factor Thresholds Used With Risk Stratification

Note that these coronary artery disease risk factors thresholds (Box 2-2) are not the same as the major risk factors for cardiovascular disease given by the American Heart Association (i.e., high blood pressure, high blood cholesterol, cigarette smoking, and phys-

---

**BOX 2-1**  **Initial ACSM Risk Stratification**

*Low risk*
Younger individuals* who are asymptomatic and meet no more than one risk factor threshold from Box 2-2

*Moderate risk*
Older individuals (men > 45 years of age; women > 55 years of age) or those who meet the threshold for two or more risk factors from Box 2-2

*High risk*
Individuals with one or more signs/symptoms listed in Box 2-3 or known cardiovascular,[†] pulmonary,[‡] or metabolic[§] disease

---

*Men < 45 years of age; women < 55 years of age.
[†] Cardiac, peripheral vascular, or cerebrovascular disease.
[‡] Chronic obstructive pulmonary disease, asthma, interstitial lung disease, or cystic fibrosis.
[§] Diabetes mellitus (types 1 and 2), thyroid disorders, renal or liver disease.

| BOX 2-2 | **Coronary Artery Disease Risk Factor Thresholds for Use With ACSM Risk Stratification***  |

| **Risk Factors** | **Defining Criteria** |
|---|---|
| *Positive* | |
| Family history | Myocardial infarction, coronary revascularization, or sudden death before 55 years of age in father or other male first-degree relative (i.e., brother or son), or before 65 years of age in mother or other female first-degree relative (i.e., sister or daughter) |
| Cigarette smoking | Current cigarette smoker or those who quit within the previous 6 months |
| Hypertension | Systolic blood pressure of 140 mmHg or diastolic 90 mmHg, confirmed by measurements on at least 2 separate occasions, or on antihypertensive medication |
| Hypercholesterolemia | Total serum cholesterol of 200 mg/dL (5.2 mmol/L) or high-density lipoprotein cholesterol of <40mg/dL (1.0 mmol/L), or on lipid-lowering medication. If low-density lipoprotein cholesterol is available, use 100 mg/dL (2.6 mmol/L) rather than total cholesterol of 200 mg/dL |
| Impaired fasting glucose | Fasting blood glucose of 110 mg/dL (6.1 mmol/L) confirmed by measurements on at least 2 separate occasions (7) |
| Obesity† | Body Mass Index of 30 kg/m$^2$, or waist girth of 100 cm |
| Sedentary lifestyle | Persons not participating in a regular exercise program or meeting the minimal physical activity recommendations‡ from the U.S. Surgeon General's report |
| *Negative* | |
| High serum HDL cholesterol§ | 60 mg/dL (1.6 mmol/L) |

*Adapted from Expert Panel on Detection, Evaluation, and Treatment of High Blood Cholesterol in Adults. National Cholesterol Education Program (NCEP) expert panel on detection, evaluation, and treatment of high blood cholesterol in adults (Adult Treatment Panel III). 2001. Note: the values used for cholesterol are different from those found in *GETP*, 6th edition, but represent the latest information from the NCEP.

†Professional opinions vary regarding the most appropriate markers and thresholds for obesity; therefore, exercise professionals should use clinical judgment when evaluating this risk factor.

‡Accumulating 30 minutes or more of moderate physical activity on most days of the week.

§It is common to sum risk factors in making clinical judgments. If high-density lipoprotein (HDL) cholesterol is high, subtract one risk factor from the sum of positive risk factors because high HDL decreases CAD risk.

ical inactivity). The intent of the ACSM coronary artery disease risk factor thresholds is for risk stratification, i.e., to make decisions regarding physician evaluation and the need for exercise testing and physician supervision requirements of the exercise test.

## Discussion of ACSM Coronary Artery Disease Risk Factor Thresholds

There are seven positive risk factors used by ACSM for risk stratification. To find a positive risk factor, simply add up the total number of risk factors that a client has or possesses.

- Family history only refers to the first degree, blood relatives of a client, such as their biological parents, siblings, and offspring. The male relative must have had a definite coronary artery disease event, such as a myocardial infarction (heart attack), coronary revascularization (e.g., bypass surgery), or sudden death from a coronary event, before age 55 years old. In female first-degree relatives, the age is before 65 years old.
- Cigarette smoking must be current, or they must have quit smoking within the last 6 months.
- Hypertension refers to having a resting blood pressure measured as equal to or above 140 mmHg systolic or equal to or above 90 mmHg diastolic, or if the client is currently taking any antihypertensive medications. Importantly, these resting blood pressures must have been assessed on at least two separate occasions.
- Hypercholesterolemia refers to having total blood cholesterol measured above 200 mg/dL or a high density lipoprotein cholesterol (HDL-C) of less than 40 mg/dL, or if the client is taking a lipid lowering medication. If the client's low density lipoprotein cholesterol (LDL-C) is known, then consider them to have hypercholesterolemia if their LDL-C is above 100 mg/dL. Similar to the hypertension risk factor threshold, if the individual is taking an antilipidemic agent, then consider them to be positive for this risk factor. While not explicitly stated in these guidelines, the measurement of cholesterol has a similar feature to the measurement of blood pressure in that it should probably be assessed on at least two separate occasions. Also, LDL-C is typically not measured but rather estimated from HDL-C and total cholesterol. Note that these values used in this test represent the latest information on high blood cholesterol from the National Cholesterol Education Program and are not the same as the values found in the 6th edition of ACSM's *GETP*.
- Impaired fasting glucose is having a fasting blood glucose (FBG) equal to or above 110 mg/dL. The FBG must also be measured and averaged on at least two separate occasions.
- Obesity is a debated risk factor threshold in terms of its definition and measurement. Thus, a fitness professional should use their clinical judgment as far as what marker to use. It is suggested by ACSM to use either the marker of a client's body mass index (BMI) or waist circumference. For this purpose, obesity may be defined as a body mass index (BMI) of greater than or equal to 30 kg/m² or a waist circumference or girth of greater than 100 cm (~40 in).
- Sedentary lifestyle is defined as a person who is not participating in a regular exercise program nor meeting the minimal recommendations of accumulating 30 minutes or more of moderate physical activity on most days of the week as set forth by the most recent report from the U.S. Surgeon General.

There is one negative risk factor used in ACSM risk stratification. If a client has or possesses this one risk factor, then subtract one from the sum of the positive risk factors.

- High serum HDL cholesterol must be above 60 mg/dL to subtract one from the sum of the positive risk factors. While it is not stated, it is important that a client have had their HDL-C measured on at least two separate occasions.

## ACSM Major Signs or Symptoms Suggestive of Cardiopulmonary Disease

There are several outward signs or symptoms that a client may have that could indicate a problem with cardiovascular, pulmonary, or metabolic (CPM) disease. These signs and symptoms can be found in Box 2-3. If a client has any of these signs or symptoms, then treat the client as high risk for ACSM risk stratification, no matter how many total ACSM coronary artery disease risk factors they may have. It is important to recognize that a physician's judgment may need to be, and should be, consulted if a client does have any of these signs or symptoms. A medical and health examination, including the HHQ, should therefore be used to evaluate for the presence of these signs or symptoms in a client. If any of these signs or symptoms are found to be present in a client then the client must be immediately referred to a physician for follow-up.

### Discussion of ACSM Major Signs or Symptoms

- Pain, discomfort (or other anginal equivalent) in the chest, neck, jaw, arms, or other areas that may be due to ischemia: Angina, also known as chest pain, is likely due to atherosclerosis or coronary artery disease. Remember that chest pain or angina is not always located in the chest of a client as it may radiate to many other locations in the body
- Shortness of breath at rest or with mild exertion: Dyspnea is the medical term and if it occurs during moderate to severe exertion it becomes somewhat less important than if it occurs while at rest or during mild exertion
- Orthopnea or paroxysmal nocturnal dyspnea: this is either difficulty with breathing when lying or sudden breathing problems at night
- Dizziness or syncope: is either a disorientated, woozy feeling or fainting episodes

---

**BOX 2-3**  **Major Signs or Symptoms Suggestive of Cardiovascular and Pulmonary Disease\***

- Pain, discomfort (or other anginal equivalent) in the chest, neck, jaw, arms, or other areas that may be due to ischemia
- Shortness of breath at rest or with mild exertion
- Dizziness or syncope
- Orthopnea or paroxysmal nocturnal dyspnea
- Ankle edema
- Palpitations or tachycardia
- Intermittent claudication
- Known heart murmur
- Unusual fatigue or shortness of breath with usual activities

\*These symptoms must be interpreted in the clinical context in which they appear because they are not all specific for cardiovascular, pulmonary, or metabolic disease.

- Ankle edema: swelling of fluid in the ankle region
- Palpitations or tachycardia: rapid throbbing or fluttering of the heart
- Intermittent claudication: severe pain in the legs when walking
- Known heart murmur: may have been previously diagnosed
- Unusual fatigue or shortness or breath with usual activities: pretty self-explanatory but it must occur with normal activities not after some strenuous task

## ACSM Recommendation for a Medical Examination and Exercise Test Based on Risk Stratification

Table 2-1 attempts to provide some recommendations concerning the need for active physician involvement with the health-related physical fitness assessment process before individualizing an exercise program for a client. As such, it is a guideline and may need to be modified based on many other issues, such as local practice or custom.

### Discussion of ACSM Recommendations

It is important to remember that Table 2-1 is a guideline for how one might want to approach pre-activity screening. For instance, a younger (< 45 years of age for men or < 55 years for women) client who is fairly healthy (meets less than two ACSM Risk Factor Thresholds) could be treated with a less strict pre-activity screening protocol (neither a medical examination nor a maximal diagnostic GXT may be necessary before starting an exercise program); however, the individual who may be a little older (> 45 for men, > 55 for women) or and/or meets 2 or more ACSM risk factor thresholds and/or has any signs or symptoms suggestive of CPM disease probably should undergo a more rigorous pre-activity screening regimen, including a medical evaluation and a diagnostic exercise test before embarking on a new exercise program.

| TABLE 2-1 | ACSM RECOMMENDATIONS FOR (A) CURRENT MEDICAL EXAMINATION* AND EXERCISE TESTING BEFORE PARTICIPATION AND (B) PHYSICIAN SUPERVISION OF EXERCISE TESTS | | |
|---|---|---|---|
| | **Low Risk** | **Moderate Risk** | **High Risk** |
| A. | | | |
| Moderate exercise[†] | Not necessary[‡] | Not necessary | Recommended |
| Vigorous exercise[§] | Not necessary | Recommended | Recommended |
| B. | | | |
| Submaximal test | Not necessary | Not necessary | Recommended |
| Maximal test | Not necessary | Recommended[‖] | Recommended |

*Within the past year (see Suggested Reading 2).
[†]Moderate exercise is defined as activities that are approximately 3 to 6 METs or the equivalent of brisk walking at 3 to 4 mph for most healthy adults (13). Nevertheless, a pace of 3 to 4 mph might be considered to be "hard" to "very hard" by some sedentary, older persons. Moderate exercise may alternatively be defined as an intensity well within the individual's capacity, one that can be comfortably sustained for a prolonged period of time (~45 min), which has a gradual initiation and progression, and is generally noncompetitive. If an individual's exercise capacity is known, relative moderate exercise may be defined by the range 40 to 60% maximal oxygen uptake.
[‡]The designation of "Not necessary" reflects the notion that a medical examination, exercise test, and physician supervision of exercise testing would not be essential in the preparticipation screening; however, they should not be viewed as inappropriate.
[§]Vigorous exercise is defined as activities of 16 METs. Vigorous exercise may alternatively be defined as exercise intense enough to represent a substantial cardiorespiratory challenge. If an individual's exercise capacity is known, vigorous exercise may be defined as an intensity of 60% maximal oxygen uptake.
[‖]When physician supervision of exercise testing is "Recommended," the physician should be in close proximity and readily available should there be an emergent need.

## ACSM Risk Stratification Case Study

The following case study is presented as an example of how to perform ACSM risk stratification:

A client decides he wants to exercise in your program. You take him through your routine pre-activity screening. He presents to you with the following information: his father died of a heart attack at the age of 52 years old. His mother was put on medication for hypertension 2 years ago at the age of 69 years. He presents no signs or symptoms of CPM disease and is a nonsmoker. He is 38 years old, he weighs 170 lbs, and is 5'8'' tall. His percent body fat was measured at 22% via skinfolds. His cholesterol is 270 mg/dL, HDL is 46 mg/dL, and his resting blood glucose is 84 mg/dL. His resting heart rate is 74 bpm and his resting blood pressure measured 132/82 and 130/84 mmHg on two separate occasions. He has a sedentary job in a factory and stands on his feet all day. He complains that as a supervisor on the job he never gets a rest throughout his shift and often is required to work overtime. He routinely plays basketball once each week with his work buddies and then goes out for few beers.

### Risk Factors Summary

| | Risk Factors | Comments |
|---|---|---|
| + | Family History | Father died of MI @ 52 yo (< 55 yo) |
| − | Cigarette Smoking | no smoking noted |
| − | Hypertension | RBP = 132/82 mmHg & 130/84 mmHg < 140/90 mmHg |
| + | Hypercholesterolemia | TC = 270 mg/dL > 200 mg/dL |
| − | Impaired Fasting Glucose | FBG =84 mg/dL < 110 mg/dL |
| − | Obesity | BMI = 25.9 kg/m$^2$ < 30 kg/m$^2$ |
| + | Sedentary Lifestyle | is not active for 30 minutes on most days |
| − | HDL | HDL = 46 mg/dL < 60 mg/dL |
| **3** | **(+) Risk Factors** | |

### Major Signs or Symptoms Suggestive of CPM Disease

None noted

### ACSM Risk Stratification

Moderate risk (has 2 or more CAD risk factors) but is young (38 years old)

### Need for Medical Examination and Exercise Testing

Could have (recommended) a medical examination and a diagnostic exercise test before starting a vigorous exercise program. All of this may not be as necessary if he is to start a moderate exercise program.

### Graded Exercise Test (GXT) Physician Supervision

A maximal exercise test, if performed, should be physician supervised (physician in close proximity and available, if needed) for this client. If performing a submaximal exercise test on him, however, physician supervision would not be necessary.

There are several case studies in Appendix B of this manual for practice with ACSM Risk Stratification.

## INFORMED CONSENT

The next step in the process of a health-related physical fitness assessment is the informed consent. Informed consent is not a form but a process we must perform for several reasons. The purpose is to inform the client about the procedures, the benefits, and the risks concerning the assessment, as well as list any of the alternatives to the assessment. The goal is to gain the client's full informed consent.

There is an example of an informed consent form in Appendix C. Two essential parts of informed consent are:

- Benefits of the particular assessment
- Risks of the particular assessment

It is through the process of listing out the risks and benefits of the assessment that we are able to demonstrate to our clients that the risk of performing the assessment is lower than the expected benefits in doing so. Also, we need to let the clients know several things about the assessment. There are at least three important things to make the client aware of before the assessment:

- The client is volunteering to participate
- The client has certain responsibilities as far as informing us of any problems they may be experiencing
- The client is free to withdraw from participation at any time with no consequences

Finally, allowing for a question and answer period from the client should complete the informed consent process.

While an example of an informed consent form is included in Appendix C of this manual, it is important to note that there are many examples of informed consent forms from several sources. It is important that while you may adopt one of these examples, you modify the form to fit your need and facility. It is also recommended that legal counsel look over the form you adopt for legal 'correctness' to the situation (e.g., facility type, etc.). Finally, it is also recommended that different informed consent forms be in place for each different component of a program (i.e., assessments and exercise programs).

## SUBJECT INTERVIEW/ORIENTATION FOR QUIET TESTS

It is common and essential to obtain a health examination and a medical history/health habits questionnaire from a client before testing. This is necessary to establish the risk for exercise and exercise testing in the client. The PAR-Q form may also be a useful tool for helping to establish the risk in individuals starting an exercise program.

The first contact most individuals have with a program is with the person who administers the subject interview/orientation. The client's impression of a program may depend on this first contact with the staff. Fitness testing is often distressing to the client and every effort should be made to allow the client to relax. Some instances will dictate more professionalism than levity so each situation must be dealt with accordingly.

The client must be informed of all the known risks and benefits of the quiet tests utilized. This is called informed consent.

### Explanation of Procedures

Describe the tests for that day: (*for example*)

- Resting Blood Pressure: "We will take (*two*) consecutive blood pressure readings while you are seated and relaxed. There will be a short relaxation period between each reading."
- Anthropometry or Body Composition: "We will estimate how much body fat you have. From this measurement we can determine an ideal weight for you. We measure body fat by *skinfolds*. We will also measure some *body girths* to give us an idea of the distribution of the body fat."

# SUBJECT INTERVIEW/ORIENTATION FOR EXERCISE TESTS

Obtain a health examination and a medical history/health habits questionnaire from the client; similar with quiet testing procedures. The PAR-Q may also be a useful tool, as previously discussed. These forms are vitally important in screening before an exercise test to make decisions concerning the level of testing and monitoring, need for supervision by physicians, and the appropriateness of testing as described in detail in ACSM's *GETP*. The client should then be informed of the risks and benefits of the exercise tests used.

## Explanation of Procedures

Describe the tests for that day: (*for example*)

- Submaximal Cycle Ergometer: "You will ride a stationary cycle at a moderate level of intensity while we record your heart rate and blood pressure response to the submaximal exercise. From this test, which may last 10 to 12 minutes, we can estimate your maximal aerobic capacity or cardiovascular fitness. This test is considered to be safe with very little risk beyond occasional leg fatigue in subjects who complete the test."
- Graded Exercise Test (GXT): "The purpose of the GXT is to find out how much exercise you can do and how your heart rate, *electrocardiogram*, and blood pressure respond to the exercise. The exercise will begin very easy (e.g., walking with no elevation or grade). The exercise will get harder and harder by increasing the speed and/or grade of the treadmill. The whole test will last between 10 to 20 minutes. We would like you to work as hard as you can. The harder you work, the more information we will have. We will, however, stop the test at your request. Your heart rate, blood pressure, and *ECG* will be monitored throughout the entire test. If we see any abnormal responses, we will stop the test and begin the cool down or recovery phase."

*Optional: (gas exchange measurement)*

"We may also measure the air you breathe out. This tells us how fit you are. From all this information, we will also be able to give you sound advice concerning your exercise habits."

Explain the risks involved in the test, but do not scare them:

- "There are some risks involved with this test. These risks range from falling on the treadmill to a heart attack, a stroke, or death, which are all rare in occurrence. *(A supervising physician may be present for the test, according to ACSM's* GETP.*)* The lab staff is trained to prevent any accidents or events, but if they do occur, we are prepared to deal with them appropriately" (in a medical setting, the risks are often stated in statistical percentages, e.g., the risk of a fatality from a GXT is generally listed as 1 in 20,000 tests).

Graded Exercise Testing; specific concerns related to the safety of the test:

- "There is a reported mortality, or death rate, of 0.5 deaths per 10,000 GXTs (1 in 20,000 GXTs). In one clinic's experience, there were no deaths in 70,000 GXTs with 6 major complications in those 70,000 tests" (more specific information can be found in ACSM's *GETP*).

Explain the post-testing procedures:

- "When you shower after the test, shower with lukewarm water, not too hot nor cold. Do not eat any heavy meals or smoke for at least 1 hour after the test. Do not exercise hard today."
- Have them sign the informed consent form to document that the process was completed. The following explanation should precede the client signing the form:
- "This form states that all the procedures have been explained to you, that you have been given the opportunity to ask questions, and that you understand the tests and risks involved. It also states that you are physically and mentally healthy for these tests. You can discontinue any test at any time. In addition, you must inform me of any and all symptoms you may develop."
- Ask them if they have any questions. If they want a copy of the informed consent form, give them one.

## EXPLANATION OF OTHER FITNESS TESTS

- Flexibility: "We will measure how far you can reach to or beyond your toes. This tells us the flexibility of your lower back and legs."
- Muscular Strength and Endurance: "We will measure your muscle strength by *having you squeeze a hand grip dynamometer as hard as you can*. We will also measure muscle endurance by having you perform (*as many sit-ups as you can in a 1 minute timed period.*)"

## SUMMARY

Pre-activity screening is a process that includes risk stratification, health appraisal, and informed consent. The process is one where the client is prepared for the upcoming physical fitness assessment. While there are several examples or models that can be followed for all of the steps of the pre-activity screening (e.g., ACSM Risk Stratification), the bottom line is the need to evaluate a client's medical readiness to undertake the health-related physical fitness assessments planned for the client. Thus, the pre-activity screening gives the assurance that the client is ready and able (based on national guidelines, such as from ACSM) to participate in the rigors of the assessment process. It is important that the fitness professional perform the pre-activity screening on their client.

## LABORATORY EXERCISES

I.  Appendix B contains several cases with all the information necessary to perform the ACSM risk stratification process.

## Suggested Readings

1. American College of Sports Medicine. ACSM's Guidelines for Exercise Testing and Prescription. 6th edition. Baltimore: Lippincott Williams & Wilkins, 2000.
2. Balady GJ, Chaitman B, Driscoll D, et al. American College of Sports Medicine and American Heart Association Joint Position Statement: Recommendations for cardiovascular screening staffing, and emergency procedures at health/fitness facilities. Med Sci Sports Exer 1998;30:1009–1018.
3. Roitman JL, ed. ACSM's Resource Manual for Guidelines for Exercise Testing and Prescription. 4th edition. Baltimore: Lippincott Williams & Wilkins, 2001.
4. Physical activity and health: a report of the Surgeon General. Atlanta, GA: U.S. Department of Health and Human Services, Centers for Disease Control and Prevention, National Center for Chronic Disease Prevention and Health Promotion, 1996.
5. Expert Panel on Detection, Evaluation, and Treatment of High Blood Cholesterol in Adults. National Cholesterol Education Program (NCEP) expert panel on detection, evaluation, and treatment of high blood cholesterol in adults (Adult Treatment Panel III). Posted on 11/19/02. http://www.nhlbi.nih.gov/guidelines/cholesterol/

# 3

# Resting and Exercise Blood Pressure and Heart Rate

## KEY TERMS

- Systolic Blood Pressure
- Diastolic Blood Pressure
- Blood Pressure Measurement: Auscultation
- Blood Pressure Measurement: Korotkoff Sounds
- Resting Heart Rate

## DEFINING BLOOD PRESSURE

*Blood pressure (BP)* is the force of blood against the walls of the arteries and veins created by the heart as it pumps blood to every part of the body. BP is typically expressed in millimeters of Mercury, mmHg. While BP is a dynamic variable with regard to location, i.e., artery versus vein and the level in an artery, we are most concerned with arterial BP at heart level. This arterial, heart-level BP is the one typically measured at rest and during exercise.

*Systolic blood pressure (SBP)* is the maximum pressure in the arteries when the ventricles contract during a heartbeat. The term derives from systole, or contraction of the heart. The SBP occurs late in ventricular systole. SBP is thought to represent the overall functioning of the left ventricle and is an important indicator of cardiovascular function during exercise. SBP is typically measured from the brachial artery at heart level and is expressed in units of millimeters of Mercury (mmHg).

*Diastolic Blood Pressure (DBP)* is the minimum pressure in the arteries when the ventricles relax. The term is derived from diastole, or relaxation of the heart. The DBP occurs late in ventricular diastole and reflects the peripheral resistance in the arterial vessels to blood flow. DBP is typically measured from the brachial artery at heart level and is expressed in units of millimeters of Mercury (mmHg).

*Hypertension*, or high BP, is a condition where the resting BP, either or both SBP and/or DBP, is chronically elevated above the optimal or desired level. The standards for classifying resting hypertension are presented later in this chapter. On the other hand, hypotension is the term for low BP. There are no accepted standards for a value for what classifies hypotension. Hypotension exists medically if the individual has symptoms related to the low BP, such as lightheadedness, dizziness, or fainting.

There are also no well-developed standards for the normal versus abnormal response of BP to exercise. A figure of the normal BP to maximal treadmill exercise is presented in this chapter.

BP is typically assessed using the principle of indirect auscultation. Auscultation is discussed further in this chapter and involves the use of a BP cuff, a manometer, and a stethoscope. Measurement of BP is a fundamental skill and is covered in detail in this chapter. In fact, the American Medical Association has stated, "... every physical educator should know how to take blood pressure and record it."

## DEFINING HEART RATE

Heart rate (HR) is the number of times that the heart contracts, usually expressed in a 1-minute time frame and reported as beats per minute (bpm). There are no known or accepted standards for resting HR. Resting HR has been thought of as an indicator of cardiovascular endurance—it tends to lower as you become more aerobically fit. There are also no standards for exercise HR, but the HR response to a standard amount of exercise is an important fitness variable and the foundation for many cardiovascular endurance tests. A figure of the normal HR response to maximal treadmill exercise is presented in this chapter. There are many ways to assess HR both at rest and during exercise including manually by palpation at various anatomical sites, use of a HR watch, or with the electrocardiogram.

## CARDIOVASCULAR HEMODYNAMICS

The cardiovascular system acts as the pump for the blood to the body with the heart serving as the pulsatile pump. The term for the overall function of the cardiovascular system is the cardiovascular hemodynamics or cardiac function. BP and HR make up some of the variables responsible for the cardiovascular hemodynamics. Cardiac output is the variable used in exercise physiology to express the overall cardiovascular hemodynamics and is related to both BP and HR.

BP and HR combined are also important indicators of cardiovascular endurance, but are not typically used as such except with clinical populations, e.g., individuals with coronary artery disease and angina pectoris (chest pain). The combination of BP and HR is known as the *rate pressure product* or *double product*. The rate pressure product is discussed further at the end of this chapter.

## MEASUREMENT OF BLOOD PRESSURE

The measurement of BP is an integral component of a resting or quiet testing physical fitness assessment session. BP measurement is a relatively simple technique. BP may be used in risk stratification as is discussed in chapter 2. Also, BP may be used in the decision about the appropriateness of performing a cardiovascular endurance test (Relative Contraindications; covered in chapter 8). The importance of BP to health and disease cannot be overemphasized. Hypertension is termed the silent killer because people with hypertension often do not recognize the condition as it typically has no symptoms. You cannot diagnose hypertension from a single measurement; serial measurements must be used on separate days. The average BP of a client should be based on the average of two or more truly resting BPs during each of two or more visits.

For accurate resting BP readings, it is important that the client be made as comfortable as possible. To accomplish this, take a few minutes to talk to the client after having them sit in a chair. Make sure the client does not have his or her legs crossed. Also, be sure to use the correct size BP cuff. There exists a White Coat Syndrome in the measurement of BP, as with many other physiological and psychological measures taken on people. This White Coat Syndrome regarding resting BP refers to an elevation of BP due to the effect of being in a doctor's office or in a clinical setting (i.e., clinician wearing a white lab coat). Thus, having a client in a relaxed state is important in resting BP measurement.

BP can be assessed indirectly via auscultation using the auscultatory method, by listening to the sounds of Korotkoff on the arterial walls. The sounds of Korotkoff are explained in detail below. The reported accuracy of indirect auscultation is within 10% of direct measures of BP made inside an artery with a pressure catheter. It is important to follow the exact procedures for the measurement of BP for accuracy.

### Theory of Auscultation

A BP cuff is applied to the upper arm or bicep region of the individual. The BP cuff is then inflated with air pressure by pumping up a hand bulb. This air pressure inside the BP cuff occludes the brachial artery of blood flow. As long as the pressure in the cuff is higher than the SBP, the artery remains occluded or collapsed and no sound is heard through the applied stethoscope in the antecubital fossa. When the artery is occluded, no blood will flow past the point of occlusion.

When the air pressure is slowly let out of the cuff, the pressure inside the cuff will eventually equal the driving pressure of the blood in the brachial artery. When the driving pressure in the artery equals the pressure inside the BP cuff, the first sound will be heard in the stethoscope. This sound is equal to the SBP.

The sounds of Korotkoff heard through the stethoscope during the BP measurement come from the turbulence of blood in the artery, which is caused by blood moving, or trying to move, from an area of higher pressure to an area of lower pressure. When the pressure inside the cuff equals the DBP, the artery is fully opened. The turbulence is no longer present and the sounds of Korotkoff disappear.

## Korotkoff Sounds

The sounds can be divided into five phases known as the sounds of Korotkoff:

*Phase 1.* SBP. The first, initial sound or the onset of sound. Sounds like: clear, repetitive tapping. This sound approximates SBP. This is the maximum pressure that occurs near the end of the stroke output or systole of the left ventricle. The SBP reflects the force of contraction of the left ventricle. The sound may be faint at first and gradually increase in intensity or volume to phase 2.

*Phase 2.* Sounds like: a soft tapping or murmur. The sounds are often longer than in the first phase. These sounds have also been described as having a swishing component. The phase 2 sounds are typically 10 to 15 mmHg after the onset of sound or below the phase 1 sounds.

*Phase 3.* Sounds like: a loud tapping sound; high in both pitch and intensity. These sounds are crisper and louder than the phase two sounds.

*Phase 4.* Also known as the TRUE DBP. Sounds like: a muffling of the sound. The sounds become less distinct and less audible. Another way of describing this sound is as soft or blowing. This is often considered the TRUE DBP, especially during exercise.

*Phase 5.* Also known as the CLINICAL DBP. Sounds like: the complete disappearance of sound. The true disappearance of sound usually occurs within 8 to 10 mmHg of the muffling of sound, also known as phase 4. Phase 5 is considered by some to be the CLINICAL DBP. This is the reading most often used for resting DBP in adults, while phase 4 is considered the TRUE DBP and should be recorded, if discerned and if significantly different from phase 5.

## Instruments Used for Blood Pressure Measurement

Sphygmomanometer: consists of a manometer and a BP cuff. The prefix sphygmo- refers to the occlusion of the artery by a cuff. A manometer is simply a device used to measure pressure. There are two common types of manometers available for BP measurement:

- Mercury
- Aneroid

Mercury is the standard for accuracy; it has the properties of being very heavy and is able to be used in a fairly small tube of ~ 350 mm (13 to 14 in) long; one can calibrate an aneroid sphygmomanometer with a mercury device. Calibration of an aneroid manometer from a mercury manometer is covered in this chapter. With the toxic nature of mercury, however, aneroid sphygmomanometers are becoming more common in the workplace. Aneroid manometers generally are used more for resting measures, while mercury manometers have been, until recently, the standard for exercise measures. Position the manometer at your eye level to eliminate the potential for any reflex errors when reading either the mercury level or the needle with the aneroid manometer. This is very important. Aneroid manometers are usually of a dial type (round) and mercury manometers are usually of a straight tube type.

Random zero sphygmomanometers exist in order to eliminate any potential bias for technicians listening for the SBP and DBP at a certain level based on their expectation of what it may likely be. With the random zero sphygmomanometer, a dial is turned by the technician before a BP measurement that changes the zero of the unit. Then the technician measures and records the BP. Finally, the technician must check on the true zero of the random zero sphygmomanometer by flipping a switch on the device to see what the zero was and subtract that value from their previously obtained SBP and DBP readings.

The cuff consists of a rubber bladder and two tubes; one to the manometer and one to a hand bulb with a valve that is used for inflation. The bladder must be of appropriate size for accurate readings. The sizing of a BP cuff should be:

- Width of bladder = 40 to 50% of arm circumference
- Length of bladder = almost long enough (~80%) to circle arm

There are three common BP cuff sizes in use in the health and fitness field: a pediatric or child cuff for small arm sizes (13 to 20 cm), a normal adult cuff for arm sizes between 24 and 32 cm, and a large adult cuff for larger arm sizes (32 to 42 cm). There are index lines on many of the newer sphygmomanometers cuffs to help 'fit' the cuff for a client's arm circumference. In general, the appropriate BP bladder should encircle at least 80% of the arm's circumference. If the cuff is too small in length or width, this will generally result in a BP that will be falsely high.

The cuff should be at the level of the heart; if below the level of the heart, then the BP reading will be falsely high. The cuff must be applied snug or tight. If the cuff is too loose, then the BP reading typically will be falsely high.

Equipment used in the measurement of BP varies greatly in its quality and is widely available commercially. BP sphygmomanometer units can be purchased in most drug stores, various health and fitness commercial catalogs, and medical supply stores. Stethoscopes are also widely available. Electric amplification of the sounds is available on some stethoscope models. As one begins to learn the skill of BP measurement or is certified in its measurement, dual head (has two sets of listening tubes/earpieces) or teaching stethoscopes are commonly used.

## Calibration of an Aneroid Sphygmomanometer

The aneroid sphygmomanometer needs to be checked for accuracy against the standard mercury sphygmomanometer on a regular (perhaps yearly) basis. This check of the accuracy, also called calibration, makes the assumption that the mercury sphygmomanometer used is accurate. Therefore, it is suggested that you use the same mercury sphygmomanometer for all calibration checks of your aneroid sphygmomanometers and that you try to limit this mercury sphygmomanometer's use to only aneroid sphygmomanometer calibration checks, if possible.

The needle on the gauge of the aneroid sphygmomanometer should rest at zero when no air pressure is inside the cuff, i.e., the air exhaust valve is all the way open and the cuff pressure has been deflated. Figure 3-1 is a drawing of the calibration setup.

1. Wrap the aneroid sphygmomanometer cuff that you are going to perform the calibration accuracy check on around a large can or bottle (similar to the circumference on the upper arm). Be sure that the aneroid gauge is readable.
2. Connect the tube from this aneroid sphygmomanometer cuff that would go to the hand bulb to one end of a "Y" connector. Note: some stethoscopes may have a "Y" connector on them so you could use that connector.
3. Connect the other end of the "Y" connector to the tube that would go from the hand bulb to the mercury sphygmomanometer you are using for the calibration accuracy check.

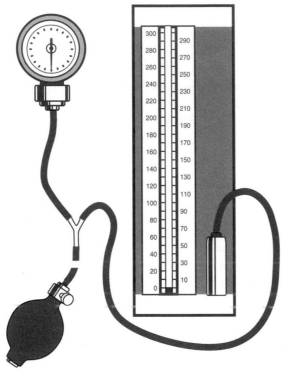

**Figure 3-1.** Line drawing of blood pressure (BP) calibration setup.

4. Connect the third end of the "Y" connector to a hand bulb. You may need to use a short piece (4 in) of extra tubing to do this.
5. Pump the hand bulb up so that a set reading is obtained on the aneroid gauge of the aneroid sphygmomanometer. For example, you may pump the aneroid cuff up to 60 mmHg.
6. Next, observe and record the level of the mercury in the mercury sphygmomanometer.
7. Deflate the bladder and repeat this procedure several more times being sure to choose some different pressures (i.e., 80, 100, 120, 140 mmHg) that coincide with the normal resting BP range.

You can now devise a mathematical correction formula specific for that aneroid sphygmomanometer based on the differences between the aneroid and mercury sphygmomanometers. For instance, if the aneroid and mercury sphygmomanometer are always off so that the mercury level always reads 4 mm more than the aneroid gauge, you then know to add 4 mmHg to every pressure recorded with that aneroid sphygmomanometer.

## PROCEDURES FOR RESTING BLOOD PRESSURE MEASUREMENT

You need to position yourself to have the best opportunity to hear the BP and see the manometer scale. Move yourself and your client to accomplish this. Take control of the client's arm, while supporting it with some piece of furniture when listening for the sounds. Make sure your stethoscope is flat and placed completely over their brachial artery. The room noise should be at a minimum and the temperature should be comfortable (70 to 74°F; 21 to 23°C). If you should have some form of sinus congestion, then your ability to hear the BP sounds may be diminished. Clearing your throat before attempting a BP measurement may be helpful. Of course, practicing the skill of resting BP measurement is important for its mastery.

Your client should be sitting, with feet flat, legs uncrossed, the arm free of any clothing, and relaxed. The arm you are using for BP measurement should be supported. Your client's back should be well supported. Measurement should begin after at least 5 full minutes of seated rest. They should be free of stimulants (nicotine products, caffeine products, alcohol, or other cardiovascular stimulants) for at least 30 minutes before the resting measurement. In addition, your client should not have exercised strenuously for at least 60 minutes.

There is no practical difference between seated and supine resting BPs, however, statistically, BP tends to be higher by about 6 to 7 mmHg for SBP and 1 mmHg for DBP in the supine position.

1. Center the rubber bladder of the BP cuff over you client's brachial artery. The lower border of cuff should be 2.5 cm (1 inch) above their antecubital fossa or crease of the elbow. Be sure to use the appropriate BP cuff, as previously discussed. Make sure you palpate your client's brachial artery as is discussed in step #5.

   It matters little which arm is chosen for the resting BP measurement; however, it is important to use the same arm for both resting and exercise measurements. The American Heart Association has recommended measuring both right and left arm BPs on your client on the initial evaluation and then choosing the arm with the higher pressure. If, however, BP is normal in the right arm, it tends to be normal in the left arm.

2. Secure the BP cuff snugly around the arm and be sure to use the appropriate sized cuff as discussed above. Your client should have no clothing on the upper arm so the cuff is properly secured. Also, clothing on the arm where you place the stethoscope will muffle the intensity of the sound.

3. Position your client's arm so it is slightly flexed at elbow; support the arm or rest it on some furniture. By having your client support the arm on a table, you can reduce the 'noise' heard during the procedure, which may increase your accuracy. Figure 3-2 below is a depiction of how the client's arm should be positioned with the BP cuff and stethoscope.

   Note: If the person does support his or her own arm, the constant isometric contraction by your client may elevate the DBP.

4. Position the BP cuff on the upper arm with the cuff at heart level.

   For every centimeter the cuff is below heart level, the BP tends to higher by 1 mmHg. The reverse is true for a BP cuff that is above heart level.

5. Find your client's brachial artery. This artery, and thus pulse, is just medial to the biceps tendon. Mark the artery with an appropriate marker (water color) to 'locate' the artery for the stethoscope bell placement. To best find your client's brachial artery, have them face the palm upwards and rotate the arm outward on the thumb side with their arm hyperextended.

6. Firmly place the bell of stethoscope over artery in antecubital fossa. Do not place the bell of the stethoscope under the lip of the BP cuff. There should be neither air space nor clothing between the bell of the stethoscope and the arm.

   The stethoscope earpieces should be facing forward, towards your nose in the same direction as your ear canal. Do not press too hard with the stethoscope bell on

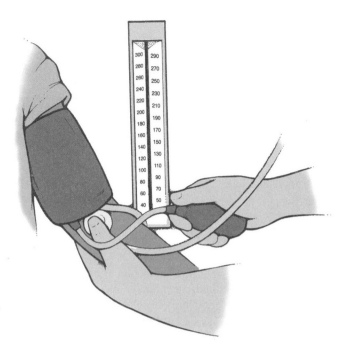

**FIGURE 3-2.** Positions of the stethoscope head and pressure cuff.

their arm. (The earpieces of a stethoscope can be cleaned between multiple users with the use of rubbing alcohol.)

7. Make sure the needle valve (air exhaust) on the hand bulb closes away from you.
    Be sure to position the manometer (either mercury or aneroid) so that the dial or tube is clearly visible and at your eye level to avoid any parallax (distortion from looking up or down) error.

8. Quickly inflate the BP cuff to about: (choose between any one of the following three accepted methods)

    • 20 mmHg above the SBP, if known (you can listen for sounds of SBP as you pump the cuff up)
    • Up to 150 to 180 mmHg, for a resting BP
    • Up to 30 mmHg above the disappearance of the radial pulse, if you palpate for radial pulse first. This is called the palpatory method (several educators favor the palpatory method when the technician is first learning BP measurement in order to 'feel' for and then listen for the SBP)

9. Deflate the pressure slowly; 2 to 3 mmHg per heartbeat (or 2 to 5 mmHg per second) by opening the air exhaust valve on the hand bulb. Rapid deflation leads to underestimation of SBP and overestimation of DBP. Slow the deflation rate to 2 mmHg per pulse beat when in the range of systolic to diastolic BP; this will compensate for slow HRs. Falsely low BPs tend to result from too fast of a deflation of the cuff.

10. Record measures of SBP and DBP (4th and 5th phase, if you can differentiate) in even numbers. Always round off upwards to the nearest 2 mmHg. Always continue to listen for any BP sounds for at least 10 mmHg below the 5th phase (to be sure you have correctly identified the 5th phase).

11. Deflate the cuff rapidly to zero after DBP is obtained.

12. Wait one full minute before redoing the BP measurement. You need to average at least two BP readings to get a 'true sense' of an individual's BP. It is suggested that you also take BP readings on your client on at least two separate occasions in order to screen for hypertension. Also, the two readings on your client in any given session should be within 5 mmHg of each other; if not you should take another BP.

## Augmentation of Sounds of Korotkoff

You may increase the intensity, or loudness, of the sounds of Korotkoff by one or more of the following methods. These methods do not increase the actual BP, just the sound level or volume.

- Pump cuff up rapidly
- Have your client raise his or her arm before you pump up the cuff
- Have your client squeeze the fist several times (~10 times) before or after pumping up the cuff

Also, be sure to rest about 1 minute between successive BP measures.

## Norms for Resting Blood Pressure

Table 3-1 presents classification standards for resting blood pressure. These norms for resting BP are for adults over the age of 18 years. To use these norms, individuals should not be taking any anti-hypertensive medications and should not be acutely ill during the measurement. When SBP and DBP fall into two different classifications, the higher classification should be selected. This classification is based on two or more readings taken at each of two or more visits after an initial BP screening. Generally, these norms are revised periodically. It is generally recommended that all persons over 30 years of age should check their BP annually.

| TABLE 3-1 | CLASSIFICATION OF RESTING BLOOD PRESSURE FOR ADULTS (AGES 18 YEARS AND OLDER)*†‡§ | |
|---|---|---|
| **Classification** | **Systolic (mmHg)** | **Diastolic (mmHg) (5ᵗʰ phase)** |
| Optimal | < 120 | < 80 |
| Normal | 120–129 | 80–84 |
| High Normal | 130–139 | 85–89 |
| Hypertension | | |
| Stage 1 (MILD) | 140–159 | 90–99 |
| Stage 2 (MODERATE) | 160–179 | 100–109 |
| Stage 3 (SEVERE) | ≥ 180 | ≥ 110 |

*Reprinted with permission from Sixth Report of the Joint Committee on Prevention, Detection, Evaluation, and Treatment of High Blood Pressure (JNC VI), Public Health Service, National Institutes of Health, National Heart, Lung and Blood Institute, NIH Publication No. 98-4080, November 1997.
†Not taking antihypertensive medication and not acutely ill. When systolic and diastolic BPs fall into different categories, the higher category should be selected to classify the individual's BP status. For example, 160/92 mmHg should be classified as stage 2 hypertension and 174/120 mmHg should be classified as stage 3 hypertension. Isolated systolic hypertension is defined as systolic BP ≥ 140 mmHg and diastolic BP < 90 mmHg and staged appropriately (e.g., 170/82 mmHg is defined as stage 2 isolated systolic hypertension). In addition to classifying stages of hypertension on the basis of average BP levels, clinicians should specify presence or absence of target organ disease and additional risk factors. This specificity is important for risk classification and treatment.
‡Optimal BP with respect to cardiovascular risk is below 120/80 mmHg. However, unusually low readings should be evaluated for clinical significance.
§Based on the average two or more readings taken at each of two or more visits after an initial screening.

# EXERCISE BLOOD PRESSURE MEASUREMENT

There is more difficulty associated with taking BPs during exercise than during rest. The technique for exercise BP measurement is not dissimilar to that used for resting BP measurement. You do need to practice this skill to master the technique. Also, exercise BP is an important physiological marker of an individual during exercise. The response of BP to exercise is an often-used criterion for test termination. Test termination criteria will be discussed further in other chapters of this manual. Also, the systolic BP is an excellent marker of left ventricular function during exercise.

A caveat concerning the measurement of exercise BP, according to the American Heart Association is: "Measurements made during exercise, as during a treadmill test, are difficult to make and often inaccurate when made with currently available equipment."

SBP should rise during aerobic exercise; either graded or steady-state, constant load exercise. However, DBP may remain the same as at rest or decline slightly. Note: individuals with large increases in SBP during a graded exercise test may be more likely to develop hypertension in the future. It is suggested that an abnormal exercise SBP response may predict future resting hypertension.

## Some Specific Suggestions for Measuring Exercise Blood Pressure

1. Secure the BP cuff to your client's arm before exercising; tape the cuff to the arm with adhesive surgical tape to keep the cuff in place. This is important considering the movement of the arm during exercise can loosen the cuff, as can sweat from the subject.
2. You should eliminate movement of the tubes that come from the cuff by being extra careful in their placement and by holding the tubes, if necessary. The tubes can bang into one another causing a sound not dissimilar from the sounds of Korotkoff. In addition, you want to try to have your client relax the arm during the measurement; any isometric contraction in your client's arm will cause fluctuations in the aneroid dial or the mercury column. Thus, it may help to grab and support your client's arm in an extended position.
3. Make sure to pump the cuff up higher than you would for a resting measurement; 180 to 200 mmHg is a reasonable starting point. As your client increases exercise intensity and the SBP rises, you may need to pump the cuff up higher; e.g. > 220 mmHg may be necessary.
4. Use an adjustable, standing manometer on wheels for the measurement of BP during exercise; these manometers can be adjusted to your eye level for easier reading and are moveable.
5. BP sounds may fall to near zero during exercise; the vibrations that cause the 5th phase can continue to low levels. Thus, the 4th sound is considered to be a better depiction of the DBP during exercise. However, both the 4th and 5th phases should be recorded, if you are able to hear a distinction between both in your client.
6. You must now concentrate and record the 4th phase sound as the true DBP during exercise. You may also record the 5th phase sound.
7. Exercise BP measurements can be difficult to hear; do not get frustrated. Keep focused on the sounds, trying to block out all other noise, and do not give up. This is an important skill. Exercise BP is generally easier to measure on a cycle as opposed to a treadmill. Also, measuring exercise BP while running on a treadmill is near impossible compared with measuring during a walking exercise.

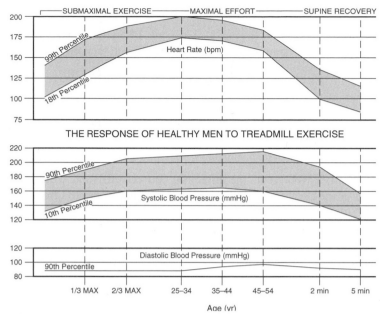

**FIGURE 3-3.** The hemodynamic responses of more than 700 healthy men to maximal treadmill exercise. Bands represent 80% of the population, with 10% having values exceeding the upper limit and 10% having lower values. (Reprinted with permission from Wolthius RA, Froelicher VF, Fischer J, et al. The response of healthy men to treadmill exercise. Circulation 1977;55:153–157.)

8. Finally, an exercise BP may take between 30 seconds to 1 minute. Thus, you need to plan ahead as far as when to take the exercise BP. It may be desirable to take the exercise BP near the start of the last minute of each stage of an exercise test.

## Norms for Exercise Blood Pressure

There are no accepted and easy to apply standards for exercise BP. Figure 3-3 and Table 3-2 detail the normal cardiovascular hemodynamics (HR and BP) response to maximal treadmill exercise.

As a side note: During cycle exercise, SBP is expected to rise, on average, about 10 to 15 mmHg for each 300 kgm · min-[1] (50 Watts) of exercise workload. Also, SBP has been shown to rise about 8 to 12 mmHg per 1 Met increase in exercise.

| | Men | | Women | |
|---|---|---|---|---|
| **TABLE 3-2** | **MEAN (+/-SD) PEAK SBP AND DBP (MMHG) DURING MAXIMAL TREADMILL EXERCISE*** | | | |
| **Age** | **SBP** | **DBP** | **SBP** | **DBP** |
| 18–29 | 182 ± 22 | 69 ± 13 | 155 ± 19 | 67 ± 12 |
| 30–39 | 182 ± 20 | 76 ± 12 | 158 ± 20 | 72 ± 12 |
| 40–49 | 186 ± 22 | 78 ± 12 | 165 ± 22 | 76 ± 12 |
| 50–59 | 192 ± 22 | 82 ± 12 | 175 ± 23 | 78 ± 11 |
| 60–69 | 195 ± 23 | 83 ± 12 | 181 ± 23 | 79 ± 11 |
| 70–79 | 191 ± 27 | 81 ± 13 | 196 ± 23 | 83 ± 11 |

*Reprinted with permission from Hiroyuki D, Allison TG, Squires RW, et al. Peak exercise blood pressure stratified by age and gender in apparently healthy subjects. Mayo Clin Proc 1996;71:445–452.

## Blood Pressure Calculations

Mean arterial pressure (MAP) is the mean, or average, BP in the arterial system. MAP represents the integration, or combination, of both the SBP and the DBP (5th phase).

$$\text{The formula for MAP} = \text{DBP} + 1/3\ (\text{SBP} - \text{DBP})$$

For example:

if SBP is 150 mmHg and DBP is 80 mmHg, then
$$\text{MAP} = 0 + 1/3\ (150 - 80)$$
$$= 103.3\ \text{mmHg}$$

Pulse pressure (PP) represents the difference between SBP and DBP. PP provides an approximation of the stroke volume (amount of blood that is ejected from the heart with each contraction).

$$\text{The formula for PP} = \text{SBP} - \text{DBP}$$

For example:

if SBP is 140 mmHg and DBP is 84 mmHg, then
$$\text{PP} = 140 - 84$$
$$= 56\ \text{mmHg}$$

## MEASUREMENT OF HEART RATE

Heart rate (HR) can be measured by several techniques; during resting or exercise including:

- Palpation of pulse at an anatomical site, such as the radial artery or carotid artery (the frequency of pulse waves per minute propagated along the peripheral arteries is usually identical to HR)
- Auscultation using a stethoscope to hear heart beat on chest (the lub-dub sound is equal to one contraction)
- Electric HR monitor/watches
- Electrocardiography (the electrical waves of depolarization and repolarization of heart cells). Electrocardiography is typically not used in health and fitness testing.

## Palpation of Pulse

There are two common anatomical sites for the measurement of HR:

- Radial: lightly press index and middle finger against the radial artery in the groove on the lateral wrist (bordered by the abductor pollicis longus and the extensor pollicis longus muscles). The radial palpation site is shown in Figure 3-4.
- Carotid: may be more visible or easily found than the radial pulse; press fingers lightly along the medial border of the sternomastoid muscle in the lower neck (on either side). Avoid the carotid sinus area (stay well below their thyroid cartilage) to avoid the reflexive slowing of HR or drop in BP by the baroreceptor reflex. The carotid palpation site is shown in Figure 3-5.

If you experience difficulty in palpating the pulse then use an HR monitor as a learning tool to check the palpated HR with the monitor's HR.

All these methods, when applied correctly, will yield similar results. The palpation of the pulse method for HR measurement should be and can be mastered through practice. However, some clients, through anatomical differences, are more difficult to palpate.

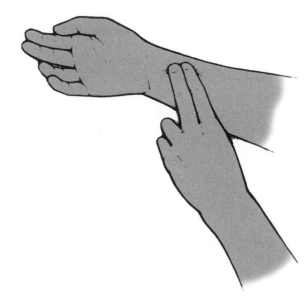

**FIGURE 3-4.** Radial artery site for heart rate measurement. From American College of Sports Medicine. ACSM's Resource Manual for Guidelines for Exercise Testing and Prescription, 4th ed. Philadelphia: Lippincott Williams & Wilkins, 2001.

## Norms for Resting Heart Rate

Of note, measuring HR by palpation of the carotid artery may lead to an underestimation of the true HR. This is because the baroreceptors in the carotid sinus region become stimulated when touched. This may reflexively reduce the client's HR as the baroreceptors sense a false increase in BP. Therefore, the radial artery is the artery of choice for palpation. Perhaps the baroreceptor reflex becomes a more important issue with HR counts longer than 15 seconds.

It is recommended that a full 60-second count be performed for accuracy in resting HR. However, a 30-second time period may be sufficient for the count. 'Resting' conditions

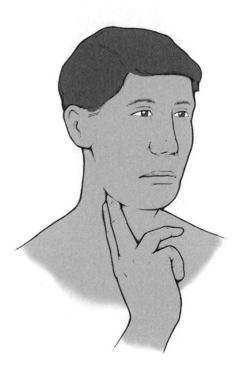

**FIGURE 3-5.** Carotid artery site for heart rate measurement. From American College of Sports Medicine. ACSM's Resource Manual for Guidelines for Exercise Testing and Prescription, 4th ed. Philadelphia: Lippincott Williams & Wilkins, 2001.

must be present (similar to resting BP). There are no known standards for resting HR classification.

## MEASUREMENT OF EXERCISE HEART RATE

By either palpation or auscultation, measure the number of beats felt or heard in a 15- or 30-second period and multiply by 4 (15 seconds) or 2 (30 seconds) to convert to a 1-minute value (bpm). The 30-second count is more accurate and less prone to error than a 15-second count. When counting the exercise HR for a time count period less than 1 minute, you should start the count at zero (reference) at the first beat felt (or heard) and start the time period at that beat. Remember, the exercise HR is an extremely important variable for many cardiovascular endurance tests.

The use of HR monitors has increased in popularity as these have become more available and affordable. Some of these monitors are prone to error, i.e., not always consistent in measuring HR; however, newer technology has resolved the reliability problem previously associated with many of these monitors. HR monitors that rely on the opacity of blood at the ear lobe or fingertip to measure/count flow are generally not as accurate as are the monitors that have a chest electrode strap.

Similar to exercise BP, there are no accepted standards for exercise HR; however, you may be able to use the normal cardiovascular hemodynamics graph for maximal treadmill exercise previously presented (Fig. 3-3). Maximal exercise HR may be important for exercise prescription with the use of the Karvonen formula (HRmax = 220 − age) and for determining if the exercise test is truly maximal and also a potential termination point for some submaximal cardiorespiratory exercise tests.

## RATE PRESSURE PRODUCT OR DOUBLE PRODUCT

The rate pressure product (RPP), or double product (DP), reflects myocardial (heart) oxygen demand or consumption ($mVO_2$). The RPP can be thought of as the heart's power output. The oxygen demand of the heart is related to the work of the heart. The RPP is the product of HR and SBP:

$$RPP = HR \cdot SBP \cdot 10^{-2}$$

The RPP is expressed in units where the resultant product is divided by 100 (10-2) to better manage the integers.

For example:

if your HR is 120 bpm and your BP is 150/90 mmHg during submaximal exercise, then
$$RPP\,(mVO_2) = 120\,bpm \cdot 150\,mmHg\,(SBP)$$
$$= 18,000$$

and then you divide by 100 ($10^{-2}$)
$$RPP\,(mVO_2) = 120 \cdot 150 \cdot 10^{-2}$$
$$= 180\,units$$

The RPP or $mVO_2$ is useful in exercise testing and training of individuals with cardiovascular disease. Often, a cardiac patient will experience angina, or chest pain, at a specific, replicable RPP or $mVO_2$. Therefore, during exercise, if the cardiac patient exceeds a certain RPP (HR and SBP combination), he or she may experience angina. Thus, when prescribing exercise for these cardiac patients, one must consider their RPP to avoid the patients experiencing angina during their exercise.

## SUMMARY

The measurement of HR and BP, both at rest and during exercise, is central to the assessment of health-related physical fitness and thus deserves its own chapter in this manual. To the fitness professional, the measurement of resting BP is one skill that is especially important to the client's overall heart health. The step-by-step approach presented in this manual should help to attain this skill through practice. Remember that practice makes perfect with most skills and so it goes with resting BP measurement.

## LABORATORY EXERCISES

1. Measure and record five subjects' BP on both their left and right sides (using their right arm and left arm) in the positions of supine (lying down), sitting, and standing. Be sure to allow for about 1 minute of rest in between BP measurements on a single subject. This exercise will allow for:

   - Measurement practice
   - Comparison between left and right sided BPs
   - Comparison between different positions (supine, sitting, standing) and BP
   - Practicing one or more of the augmentation procedures to help hearing the Korotkoff sounds.

2. Measure and record three subject's HR and BP response to exercise. Have the subject exercise on a stationary cycle ergometer (Monark brand [Vansbro, Sweden] preferably). First, measure the resting HR and BP. Next, have the subject cycle at 50 Watts (300 kpm/min) for 5 minutes (measure their exercise HR and BP during the last minute of exercise). Have the subject continue to cycle at 100 watts (600 kpm/min) for another 5 minutes while you record the HR and BP in the last minute of that stage. (There is more information on stationary cycle workloads in chapter 7.)

   - This exercise should allow you to make comparisons between the HR and BP response to exercise (resting to moderate exertion).
   - Be sure to listen to and record the 4th and 5th Korotkoff sounds.

### Suggested Readings

1. Sixth Report of the Joint Committee on Prevention, Detection, Evaluation, and Treatment of High Blood Pressure (JNCVI), Public Health Service, National Institutes of Health, National Heart, Lung and Blood Institute, NIH Publication No. 98-4080, November 1997.
2. Prisant LM, Alpert BS, Robbins CB, et al. American national standard for nonautomated sphygmomanometry. American J Hypertension 1995;8:210–213.
3. Perloff D, Grimm C, Flack J, et al. Human blood pressure determination by sphygmomanometry. Circulation.1993;88 (5 part 1):2460–2470.

# 4

# Body Composition

## DEFINING BODY COMPOSITION

Body composition is defined as the relative proportion of fat and fat-free tissue in the body. The assessment of body composition is necessary for a variety of reasons. There is a strong correlation between obesity and an increased risk of a variety of chronic diseases (coronary artery disease [CAD], diabetes, hypertension, certain cancers, hyperlipidemia). Assessing body composition can be helpful for establishing optimal weight for health and physical performance.

The following terms should not be used interchangeably.

- *Overweight* is generally defined as a deviation in body weight from some standard or "ideal" weight in relation to height. In large surveys, desirable weight is established as the weight (or weight range) associated with the lowest mortality. The 1983 Metropolitan Life Insurance Table is one example of such a national survey (Table 4-1). Frame size, by elbow breadth, has been considered in more recent tables to increase the applicability of the height-weight tables or charts. The most common standard that is accepted in the literature defines overweight as 20% above ideal weight. Overweight does not always reflect obesity (athletes can be lean but over their ideal body weight).

- *Overfat* is desirable percent body fat that has been expressed several different ways in the literature. Differences in the desirable percent body fat ranges exist for men and women: the concept of essential body fat is generally about 2 to 3% in men; gender-specific body fat for female reproduction is generally about 8 to 12% for women.

- *Obesity* can be defined as a surplus of adipose tissue resulting from excessive energy intake relative to energy expenditure. Excessive weight is associated with an increased risk of mortality and morbidity, including coronary artery disease, hypertension, non-insulin dependent diabetes, and other illnesses. Obesity is a major public health concern in the United States with over 97 million Americans either overweight or obese.

## HEALTH IMPLICATIONS OF OBESITY

Increased morbidity and mortality are associated with obesity. The famous 'J-shaped' curve of mortality and Body Mass Index (BMI) represent this relationship where both the very lean, or underweight, and the obese, experience the highest mortality. Meanwhile, those individuals of moderate weight or body build have the lowest mortality (Fig. 4-1).

Some of the chronic diseases that have a strong association with obesity are:

- Coronary artery disease (CAD)
- Hypertension (HTN)
- Non-insulin-dependent diabetes mellitus (NIDDM)
- Hyperlipemia (high blood cholesterol)
- Certain cancers

## ANTHROPOMETRY—BODY COMPOSITION

*Anthropometry* is the measurement of the human body. Several techniques fall into this category: height/weight, circumferences/girths, and skinfolds. Different anthropometric measurement techniques employ a variety of measurement sites and instruments. Some of these techniques (such as skinfold assessment) are estimations of body composition or body fat, while other techniques (such as BMI) are assessments of body build.

## TABLE 4-1  SUGGESTED BODY WEIGHTS FOR ADULTS

### A. NATIONAL INSTITUTES OF HEALTH RECOMMENDATIONS

| Height[1] | Weight in Pounds[2] | |
|---|---|---|
| | 19 to 34 y | 35 y+ |
| 5'0" | 97–128 | 108–138 |
| 5'1" | 101–132 | 111–143 |
| 5'2" | 104–137 | 115–148 |
| 5'3" | 107–141 | 119–152 |
| 5'4" | 111–146 | 122–157 |
| 5'5" | 114–150 | 126–162 |
| 5'6" | 118–155 | 130–167 |
| 5'7" | 121–160 | 134–172 |
| 5'8" | 125–164 | 138–178 |
| 5'9" | 129–169 | 142–183 |
| 5'10" | 132–174 | 146–188 |
| 5'11" | 136–179 | 151–194 |
| 6'0" | 140–184 | 155–199 |
| 6'1" | 144–189 | 159–205 |
| 6'2" | 148–195 | 164–210 |
| 6'3" | 152–200 | 168–216 |
| 6'4" | 156–205 | 173–222 |
| 6'5" | 160–211 | 177–228 |
| 6'6" | 164–216 | 182–234 |

[1]Without shoes
[2]Without clothes
(From *Understanding Adult Obesity,* National Institute of Diabetes and Digestive and Kidney Diseases. National Institutes of Health, U.S. Department of Health and Human Services)

### C. HOW TO DETERMINE FRAME SIZE

The person's right arm extends forward perpendicular to the body, with the arm bent so the angle at the elbows forms 90° with the fingers pointing up and the palm turned away from the body. The greatest breadth across the elbow joint is measured with a sliding caliper along the axis of the upper arm, on the two prominent bones on either side of the elbow. This breadth represents elbow breadth. The following give the elbow breadth measurements for medium-framed men and women of various heights. Measurements lower than those listed indicate a small frame size; higher measurements indicate a large frame size.

| Men | | Women | |
|---|---|---|---|
| **Height 1 Heels** | **Elbow Breadth** | **Height 2 Heels** | **Elbow Breadth** |
| 5'2"–5'3" | 2 1/2"–2 7/8" | 4'10"–4'11" | 2 1/4"–2 1/2" |
| 5'4"–5'7" | 2 5/8"–2 7/8" | 5'0"–5'3" | 2 1/4"–2 1/2" |
| 5'8"–5'11" | 2 3/4"–3" | 5'4"–5'7" | 2 3/8"–2 5/8" |
| 6'0"–6'3" | 2 3/4"–3 1/8" | 5'8"–5'11" | 2 3/8"–2 5/8" |
| > 6'4" | 2 7/8"–3 1/4" | ≥ 6'0" | 2 1/2"–2 3/4" |

From Metropolitan Life Insurance Company, 1983.

### B. 1983 METROPOLITAN LIFE INSURANCE HEIGHT-WEIGHT TABLE*

| Men | | | | | Women | | | |
|---|---|---|---|---|---|---|---|---|
| **Height Ft.  In.** | | **Small Frame** | **Medium Frame** | **Large Frame** | **Height Ft.  In.** | | **Small Frame** | **Medium Frame** | **Large Frame** |
| 5' | 2" | 128–134 | 131–141 | 138–150 | 4' | 10" | 102–111 | 109–121 | 118–131 |
| 5' | 3" | 130–136 | 133–143 | 140–153 | 4' | 11" | 103–113 | 111–123 | 120–134 |
| 5' | 4" | 132–138 | 135–145 | 142–156 | 5' | 0" | 104–115 | 113–126 | 122–137 |
| 5' | 5" | 134–140 | 137–148 | 144–160 | 5' | 1" | 106–118 | 115–129 | 125–140 |
| 5' | 6" | 136–142 | 139–151 | 146–164 | 5' | 2" | 108–121 | 118–132 | 128–143 |
| 5' | 7" | 138–145 | 142–154 | 149–168 | 5' | 3" | 111–124 | 121–135 | 131–147 |
| 5' | 8" | 140–148 | 145–157 | 152–172 | 5' | 4" | 114–127 | 124–138 | 134–151 |
| 5' | 9" | 142–151 | 148–160 | 155–176 | 5' | 5" | 117–130 | 127–141 | 137–155 |
| 5' | 10" | 144–154 | 151–163 | 158–180 | 5' | 6" | 120–133 | 130–144 | 140–159 |
| 5' | 11" | 146–157 | 154–166 | 161–184 | 5' | 7" | 123–136 | 133–147 | 143–163 |
| 6' | 0" | 149–160 | 157–170 | 164–188 | 5' | 8" | 126–139 | 136–150 | 146–167 |
| 6' | 1" | 152–164 | 160–174 | 168–192 | 5' | 9" | 129–142 | 139–153 | 149–170 |
| 6' | 2" | 155–168 | 164–178 | 172–197 | 5' | 10" | 132–145 | 142–156 | 152–173 |
| 6' | 3" | 158–172 | 167–182 | 176–202 | 5' | 11" | 135–148 | 145–159 | 155–176 |
| 6' | 4" | 162–176 | 171–187 | 181–207 | 6' | 0" | 138–151 | 148–162 | 158–179 |

*Weights at ages 25–59 y based on lowest comparative mortality. Weight in lb according to frame size for men wearing indoor clothing weighing 5 lb, shoes with 1-in. heels; for women, indoor clothing, shoes 2-in. heels. From *Statistical Bulletin,* Metropolitan Life Insurance Company, New York City.

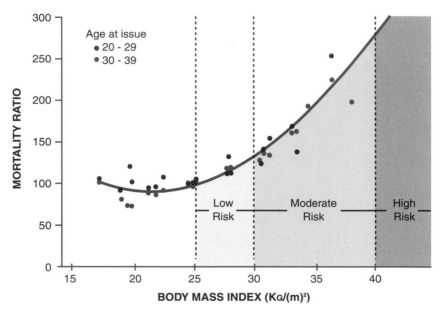

**Figure 4-1.** Relation of BMI and mortality.

There is a frequent need to evaluate body weight and composition in the health and fitness field. Most often this is done to establish a target, desirable, or optimal weight for an individual. There are several ways to evaluate the composition of the human body. Body composition can be estimated with both laboratory and field techniques that vary in terms of complexity, cost, and accuracy. One of the most accurate means of assessing body composition is by hydrostatic weighing. Hydrostatic weighing, also known as underwater weighing, is often considered a criterion standard for assessing body composition.

Although underwater weighing is simple in theory, it generally requires expensive laboratory equipment and is inconvenient for the subject; therefore, this technique is not widely used. The health and fitness field relies on other methods of anthropometry in the assessment of body build, body composition, and obesity. The following techniques will be reviewed:

- Height and weight
- Body Mass Index
- Waist-to-hip ratio
- Girths/circumference
- Skinfolds
- Bioelectrical impedance analysis
- Hydrostatic weighing

Selecting the appropriate technique is based on the relative precision, reliability, and accuracy of available methods and equations. Table 4-2 can be used as a guide to selecting an appropriate method to assess body composition on your client. Each of these techniques will be discussed further in this manual.

| TABLE 4-2 | RATINGS OF THE VALIDITY AND OBJECTIVITY OF BODY COMPOSITION METHODS |

| Method | Precision | Objectivity | Accuracy | Valid Equations | Overall |
|---|---|---|---|---|---|
| Body mass index | 1 | 1 | 4, 5 | 4,5 | 4 |
| Near infrared interactance | 1 | 1, 2 | 4 | 4 | 3.5 |
| Skinfolds | 2 | 2, 3 | 2, 3 | 2, 3 | 2.5 |
| Bioelectric impedance | 2 | 2 | 2, 3 | 2, 3 | 2.5 |
| Circumferences | 2 | 2 | 2, 3 | 2, 4 | 3.0 |

1, excellent; 2, very good; 3, good; 4, fair; 5, unacceptable.
Precision is reliability within investigators; objectivity is reliability between investigators; accuracy refers to comparison with a criterion method; valid equations are cross-validated.

## Procedures for Height and Weight

1. Measure the height of the subject. With shoes removed, instruct the subject to stand straight up, take a deep breath and hold it, and look straight ahead. Record the height of the subject in centimeters or inches.

   1 in = 2.54 cm
   1 m = 100 cm
   For example: 6 ft = 72 in = 183 cm = 1.83 m

2. Weigh the subject with the shoes and as much other clothing removed as possible. Convert the resulting weight from pounds to kilograms.

   1 kg = 2.2 lbs
   For example: 187 lbs = 85 kg

3. Next, compare the subject's height and weight to the 1983 Height/Weight Table by Metropolitan Life Insurance (Table 4-1). Note: the height/weight tables have several deficiencies, including using a select group of individuals for development (e.g., people who purchase life insurance) and the imprecise concept of 'frame size.'

## Body Mass Index (BMI)

Body mass index (BMI), also called the Quetelet's Index, is used to assess weight relative to height. BMI has a similar association with body fat as the height-weight tables previously discussed. This technique compares an individual's weight (in kilograms) to their height (in meters, squared), much like a height/weight table would. The BMI gives a single number for comparison, as opposed to the weight to height ranges on the tables.

One popular formula for BMI is:

$$\text{Body Mass Index (kg} \cdot \text{m}^{-2}) = \frac{\text{WT (kg)}}{\text{HT (m}^2)}$$

For example:
   Figure the BMI for an individual who weighs 150 lbs and is 5'8".
   5'8" = 173 cm = 1.73 m = $1.73^2$ = 2.99
   and 150 lbs = 68 kg

$$\text{BMI} = \frac{68}{2.99} = 22.7 \text{ kg} \cdot \text{m}^{-2}$$

**TABLE 4-3** CLASSIFICATION OF DISEASE RISK BASED ON BODY MASS INDEX (BMI) AND WAIST CIRCUMFERENCE*

| | BMI, kg/m² | Disease Risk† Relative to Normal Weight and Waist Circumference‡ | |
| --- | --- | --- | --- |
| | | Men, ≤102 cm; Women, ≤88 cm | Men, >102 cm; Women, >88 cm |
| Underweight | <18.5 | ... | ... |
| Normal§ | 18.5–24.9 | ... | ... |
| Overweight | 25.0–29.9 | Increased | High |
| Obesity, class | | | |
| I | 30.0–34.9 | High | Very high |
| II | 35.0–39.9 | Very high | Very high |
| III | ≥40 | Extremely high | Extremely high |

*Modified from Expert Panel. Executive summary of the clinical guidelines on the identification, evaluation, and treatment of overweight and obesity in adults. Arch Intern Med 1998;158:1855–1867.
†Disease risk for type 2 diabetes, hypertension, and cardiovascular disease. Ellipses indicate that no additional risk at these levels of BMI was assigned.
‡A gender neutral value for waist circumference (>100 cm) has also been suggested as an index of obesity (see Box 2-2).
§Increased waist circumference can also be a marker for increased risk even in persons of normal weight.

The major problem with using BMI for body composition is that it is difficult for a client to interpret weight loss or gain. The BMI does not differentiate fat weight from fat-free weight. BMI has only a modest correlation with percent body fat predicted from hydrostatic weighing. BMI does represent an improvement over the relationship between only weight and percent body fat. Figure 4-1 demonstrates the relationship between BMI and disease risk.

## Waist-to-Hip Ratio (WHR)

The waist-to-hip ratio is a comparison between the circumference of the waist to the circumference of the hip. This ratio best represents the distribution of body weight, and perhaps body fat, on an individual. The pattern of body weight distribution is recognized as an important predictor of health risks of obesity. Individuals with more weight or circumference on the trunk are at increased risk of hypertension, type 2 diabetes, hyperlipidemia, and CAD compared to individuals who are of equal weight but have more of their weight distributed on the extremities. Some experts suggest that the waist circumference alone may be used as an indicator of health risk (Table 4-3).

- Waist: The waist circumference is frequently defined as the smallest waist circumference usually above the umbilicus or navel (1 inch above umbilicus; below the xiphoid process) (Fig. 4-2).
- Hip: In the studies that have assessed WHR, the hip circumference is defined as the largest circumference around the buttocks, above the gluteal fold (posterior extension) (Fig. 4-3).

The WHR also may be expressed, or used interchangeably, as the A:G ratio. The A:G ratio stands for abdominal to gluteal ratio. WHR is expressed as a ratio (there are no units).

$$\text{WHR} = \frac{\text{Waist Circumference}}{\text{Hip Circumference}}$$

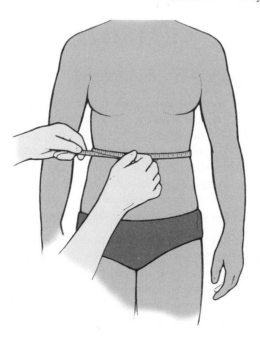

**FIGURE 4-2.** Waist circumference.

Measure the waist and hip circumferences in either inches or centimeters (1 in = 2.54 cm). Take multiple measurements until each is within ¼ inch of each other.

For example:

A male client has a waist circumference of 32 in (81.3 cm) and a hip circumference of 35 in (86.4 cm). The WHR is $^{32}/_{35}$ = 0.914 (0.91)

An increased risk of overall mortality is associated with upper body obesity. A person with upper body obesity is carrying more weight on the trunk compared to the buttocks and has a higher WHR than lower body obesity. The waist circumference may

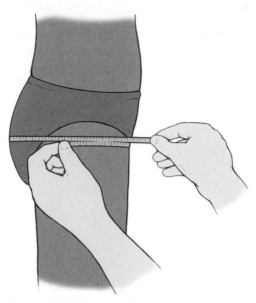

**FIGURE 4-3.** Hip circumference.

also be used alone as an indicator of abdominal obesity. See Table 4-4 for normative data on WHR.

## Circumferences (Girths)

Circumferences have been used for many years in the estimation of body composition. Circumferences have the advantages of being easily learned, quick to administer, and inexpensive in equipment needs. Circumferences, also known as girths, can also be used to measure muscle girth size and, therefore, quantify changes in muscle with specific training (e.g., resistance weight training). Perhaps the most important application of circumferences is its ease in documenting changes in body size (e.g., a reduction in waist size with weight loss efforts). Also, some body composition formulas use a combination of circumference and skinfold measurements in estimating the percentage of body fat.

1. Read the circumference (girth) to the nearest half of a centimeter (5 mm). Apply the tape to the site so it is taut but not tight. Avoid skin compression or pinching of the skin. Take at least duplicate measures at each site and average the measurements (duplicate measurements should be within 7 mm). Many available tapes have a spring mechanism that guides you in how taut to pull the tape (a Gulick-type tape may be used to ensure that the tape is taut). Using a quality tape is important; a steel tape is best, but a plastic tape may suffice.
2. The subject should stand straight or erect but relaxed (including all body parts, like the biceps) at all times.
3. Be sure to use standardized sites for measurement. This circumference estimation of percent body fat uses 3 circumference sites that are specific to the subject's gender and age group, as follows:

### Specific Circumference Sites by Gender and Age Group

* Young men (18–26 years of age): Right upper arm, abdomen, and right forearm
* Young women (18–26 years of age): Abdomen, right thigh, and right forearm
* Older men (27–50 years of age): Buttocks, abdomen, and right forearm
* Older women (27–50 years of age): Abdomen, right thigh, and right calf

**TABLE 4-4    WAIST-TO-HIP CIRCUMFERENCE RATIO (WHR) STANDARD FOR MEN AND WOMEN**

|  | Age | Risk Low | Moderate | High | Very High |
|---|---|---|---|---|---|
| Men | 20–29 | <0.83 | 0.83–0.88 | 0.89–0.94 | >0.94 |
|  | 30–39 | <0.84 | 0.84–0.91 | 0.92–0.96 | >0.96 |
|  | 40–49 | <0.88 | 0.88–0.95 | 0.96–1.00 | >1.00 |
|  | 50–59 | <0.90 | 0.90–0.96 | 0.97–1.02 | >1.02 |
|  | 60–69 | <0.91 | 0.91–0.98 | 0.99–1.03 | >1.03 |
| Women | 20–29 | <0.71 | 0.71–0.77 | 0.78–0.82 | >0.82 |
|  | 30–39 | <0.72 | 0.72–0.78 | 0.79–0.84 | >0.84 |
|  | 40–49 | <0.73 | 0.73–0.79 | 0.80–0.87 | >0.87 |
|  | 50–59 | <0.74 | 0.74–0.81 | 0.82–0.88 | >0.88 |
|  | 60–69 | <0.76 | 0.76–0.83 | 0.84–0.90 | >0.90 |

(Reprinted with permission from Heyward VH, Stolarczyk LM. Applied Body Composition Assessment. Champaign, IL: Human Kinetics, 1996:82).

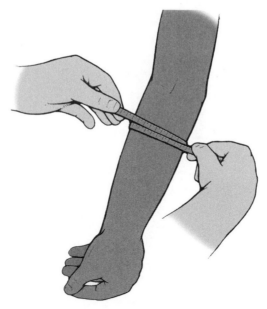

**FIGURE 4-4.** Forearm circumference.

## Circumference Anatomical Sites

The anatomical sites for circumference measurements are:

- Right forearm: maximum girth around the lower arm or forearm with the right arm straight, extended in front of the body, and the palm up (Fig. 4-4).
- Right upper arm or biceps: midpoint between shoulder and elbow with the right arm straight, extended in front of body, and the palm up (Fig. 4-5).
- Abdomen (waist): a horizontal line 1 inch above the umbilicus (navel) or at the smallest circumference in this area (below the rib cage). Measurement is taken at end of a normal expiration.
- Buttocks (hips or gluteal): the largest horizontal plane around the buttocks. Subject should have their heels together.

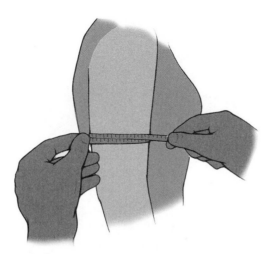

**FIGURE 4-5.** Upper arm circumference.

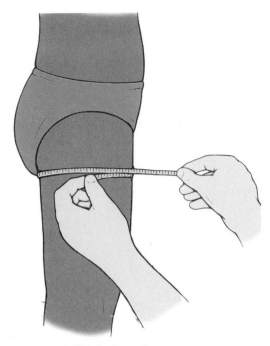

**FIGURE 4-6.** Thigh circumference.

- Right thigh (proximal thigh): the upper right thigh, just below the buttocks (gluteal fold) at the maximal circumference with the legs slightly apart (Fig. 4-6).
- Right calf: the largest horizontal plane on the right calf, usually midway between knee and ankle (Fig. 4-7).

Note: There is considerable variability among experts as to the exact anatomical site and terminology for the waist and abdominal sites. The descriptions above refer to the

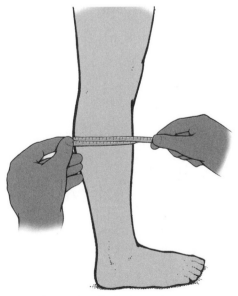

**FIGURE 4-7.** Calf circumference.

waist and abdomen site as being the same. Some experts separate these into two distinct sites: abdominal (level of umbilicus, usually larger than waist) and waist (smallest circumference around the torso; usually 1–2 inches above umbilicus).

Use the age- and gender-specific charts provided to predict percent body fat from circumference measures. Convert the measurement taken at the particular site to its constant found in Table 4-5. The formulas for percent body fat are:

| | |
|---|---|
| Young Men: | Constant A + B − C − 10.2 = % Body Fat |
| Young Women: | Constant A + B − C − 19.6 = % Body Fat |
| Older Men: | Constant A + B − C − 15.0 = % Body Fat |
| Older Women: | Constant A + B − C − 18.4 = % Body Fat |

For example:

If a 22-year-old man has the following circumference measurements, then his percent body fat would be:

| Site | Measurement (cm) | Constant |
|---|---|---|
| Right upper arm: | 40 | 58.29 |
| Abdomen: | 73 | 37.37 |
| Right forearm: | 27 | 58.37 |

| Constant A | + | Constant B | − Constant C | − 10.2 = % Body Fat |
|---|---|---|---|---|
| 58.29 | + | 37.37 | − 58.37 | − 10.2 = 27.09% (27.1) |

## Skinfold Determination

Skinfold determination of percent body fat can be quite accurate when performed by a properly trained technician with skinfold calipers. It should be remembered, however, that skinfold determination of percent body fat is still an estimate or prediction of percent body fat, not an absolute measurement. This estimate is based on the principle that the amount of subcutaneous fat is proportional to the total amount of body fat; however, the proportion of subcutaneous to total fat varies with gender, age, and ethnicity. Regression equations considering these factors have been developed to predict body density or percent fat from skinfold measurements. The American College of Sports Medicine (Box 4-1) provides specific recommendations for standardizing anatomical sites (Fig. 4-8).

The following procedures may help standardize the measure:

1. Firmly grasp a double fold of skin (a skinfold) and the subcutaneous fat between the thumb and index finger of your left hand and lift up away from the body. Be certain that you have not grasped any muscle and that you have taken up all the fat. It may be helpful to roll the skinfold between your two fingers to ensure this. You can also have the subject first flex the muscle below the site to help identify muscle from fat before you measure. Be sure, however, to have the subject relax the area before taking the measurement.

2. You should grasp the skinfold site with your two fingers about 8 cm (3 in) apart on a line that is perpendicular to the long axis of the skinfold site. You should be able to form a fold that has roughly parallel sides. Larger skinfolds (obese individuals) will require you to separate your fingers further than 8 cm.

3. Hold the caliper in your right hand with the scale facing up to ease your viewing. Place the contact surfaces of the caliper 1 cm (0.5 in) below your fingers. The calipers should be placed on the exact skinfold site, while your fingers should be

(*text continues on page 62*)

**TABLE 4-5   CONVERSION CONSTANTS TO PREDICT PERCENT BODY FAT
FOR YOUNG MEN[A]**

| Upper Arm | | | Abdomen | | | Forearm | | |
|---|---|---|---|---|---|---|---|---|
| in | cm | Constant A | in | cm | Constant B | in | cm | Constant C |
| 7.00 | 17.78 | 25.91 | 21.00 | 53.34 | 27.56 | 7.00 | 17.78 | 38.01 |
| 7.25 | 18.41 | 26.83 | 21.25 | 53.97 | 27.88 | 7.25 | 18.41 | 39.37 |
| 7.50 | 19.05 | 27.76 | 21.50 | 54.61 | 28.21 | 7.50 | 19.05 | 40.72 |
| 7.75 | 19.68 | 28.68 | 21.75 | 55.24 | 28.54 | 7.75 | 19.68 | 42.08 |
| 8.00 | 20.32 | 29.61 | 22.00 | 55.88 | 28.87 | 8.00 | 20.32 | 43.44 |
| 8.25 | 20.95 | 30.53 | 22.25 | 56.51 | 29.20 | 8.25 | 20.95 | 44.80 |
| 8.50 | 21.59 | 31.46 | 22.50 | 57.15 | 29.52 | 8.50 | 21.59 | 46.15 |
| 8.75 | 22.22 | 32.38 | 22.75 | 57.78 | 29.85 | 8.75 | 22.22 | 47.51 |
| 9.00 | 22.86 | 33.31 | 23.00 | 58.42 | 30.18 | 9.00 | 22.86 | 48.87 |
| 9.25 | 23.49 | 34.24 | 23.25 | 59.05 | 30.51 | 9.25 | 23.49 | 50.23 |
| 9.50 | 24.13 | 35.16 | 23.50 | 59.69 | 30.84 | 9.50 | 24.13 | 51.58 |
| 9.75 | 24.76 | 36.09 | 23.75 | 60.32 | 31.16 | 9.75 | 24.76 | 52.94 |
| 10.00 | 25.40 | 37.01 | 24.00 | 60.96 | 31.49 | 10.00 | 25.40 | 54.30 |
| 10.25 | 26.03 | 37.94 | 24.25 | 61.59 | 31.82 | 10.25 | 26.03 | 55.65 |
| 10.50 | 26.67 | 38.86 | 24.50 | 62.23 | 32.15 | 10.50 | 26.67 | 57.01 |
| 10.75 | 27.30 | 39.79 | 24.75 | 62.86 | 32.48 | 10.75 | 27.30 | 58.37 |
| 11.00 | 27.94 | 40.71 | 25.00 | 63.50 | 32.80 | 11.00 | 27.94 | 59.73 |
| 11.25 | 28.57 | 41.64 | 25.25 | 64.13 | 33.13 | 11.25 | 28.57 | 61.08 |
| 11.50 | 29.21 | 42.56 | 25.50 | 64.77 | 33.46 | 11.50 | 29.21 | 62.44 |
| 11.75 | 29.84 | 43.49 | 25.75 | 65.40 | 33.79 | 11.75 | 29.84 | 63.80 |
| 12.00 | 30.48 | 44.41 | 26.00 | 66.04 | 34.12 | 12.00 | 30.48 | 65.16 |
| 12.25 | 31.11 | 45.34 | 26.25 | 66.67 | 34.44 | 12.25 | 31.11 | 66.51 |
| 12.50 | 31.75 | 46.26 | 26.50 | 67.31 | 34.77 | 12.50 | 31.75 | 67.87 |
| 12.75 | 32.38 | 47.19 | 26.75 | 67.94 | 35.10 | 12.75 | 32.38 | 69.23 |
| 13.00 | 33.02 | 48.11 | 27.00 | 68.58 | 35.43 | 13.00 | 33.02 | 70.59 |
| 13.25 | 33.65 | 49.04 | 27.25 | 69.21 | 35.76 | 13.25 | 33.65 | 71.94 |
| 13.50 | 34.29 | 49.96 | 27.50 | 69.85 | 36.09 | 13.50 | 34.29 | 73.30 |
| 13.75 | 34.92 | 50.89 | 27.75 | 70.48 | 36.41 | 13.75 | 34.92 | 74.66 |
| 14.00 | 35.56 | 51.82 | 28.00 | 71.12 | 36.74 | 14.00 | 35.56 | 76.02 |
| 14.25 | 36.19 | 52.74 | 28.25 | 71.75 | 37.07 | 14.25 | 36.19 | 77.37 |
| 14.50 | 36.83 | 53.67 | 28.50 | 72.39 | 37.40 | 14.50 | 36.83 | 78.73 |
| 14.75 | 37.46 | 54.59 | 28.75 | 73.02 | 37.73 | 14.75 | 37.46 | 80.09 |
| 15.00 | 38.10 | 55.52 | 29.00 | 73.66 | 38.05 | 15.00 | 38.10 | 81.45 |
| 15.25 | 38.73 | 56.44 | 29.25 | 74.29 | 38.38 | 15.25 | 38.73 | 82.80 |
| 15.50 | 39.37 | 57.37 | 29.50 | 74.93 | 38.71 | 15.50 | 39.37 | 84.16 |
| 15.75 | 40.00 | 58.29 | 29.75 | 75.56 | 39.04 | 15.75 | 40.00 | 85.52 |
| 16.00 | 40.64 | 59.22 | 30.00 | 76.20 | 39.37 | 16.00 | 40.64 | 86.88 |
| 16.25 | 41.27 | 60.14 | 30.25 | 76.83 | 39.69 | 16.25 | 41.27 | 88.23 |
| 16.50 | 41.91 | 61.07 | 30.50 | 77.47 | 40.02 | 16.50 | 41.91 | 89.59 |
| 16.75 | 42.54 | 61.99 | 30.75 | 78.10 | 40.35 | 16.75 | 42.54 | 90.95 |
| 17.00 | 43.18 | 62.92 | 31.00 | 78.74 | 40.68 | 17.00 | 43.18 | 92.31 |
| 17.25 | 43.81 | 63.84 | 31.25 | 79.37 | 41.01 | 17.25 | 43.81 | 93.66 |
| 17.50 | 44.45 | 64.77 | 31.50 | 80.01 | 41.33 | 17.50 | 44.45 | 95.02 |
| 17.75 | 45.08 | 65.69 | 31.75 | 80.64 | 41.66 | 17.75 | 45.08 | 96.38 |

*(continued)*

## TABLE 4-5  CONVERSION CONSTANTS TO PREDICT PERCENT BODY FAT FOR YOUNG MEN[a] *(Continued)*

| Upper Arm | | | Abdomen | | | Forearm | | |
|---|---|---|---|---|---|---|---|---|
| in | cm | Constant A | in | cm | Constant B | in | cm | Constant C |
| 18.00 | 45.72 | 66.62 | 32.00 | 81.28 | 41.99 | 18.00 | 45.72 | 97.74 |
| 18.25 | 46.35 | 67.54 | 32.25 | 81.91 | 42.32 | 18.25 | 46.35 | 99.09 |
| 18.50 | 46.99 | 68.47 | 32.50 | 82.55 | 42.65 | 18.50 | 46.99 | 100.45 |
| 18.75 | 47.62 | 69.40 | 32.75 | 83.18 | 42.97 | 18.75 | 47.62 | 101.81 |
| 19.00 | 48.26 | 70.32 | 33.00 | 83.82 | 43.30 | 19.00 | 48.26 | 103.17 |
| 19.25 | 48.89 | 71.25 | 33.25 | 84.45 | 43.63 | 19.25 | 48.89 | 104.52 |
| 19.50 | 49.53 | 72.17 | 33.50 | 85.09 | 43.96 | 19.50 | 49.53 | 105.88 |
| 19.75 | 50.16 | 73.10 | 33.75 | 85.72 | 44.29 | 19.75 | 50.16 | 107.24 |
| 20.00 | 50.80 | 74.02 | 34.00 | 86.36 | 44.61 | 20.00 | 50.80 | 108.60 |
| 20.25 | 51.43 | 74.95 | 34.25 | 86.99 | 44.94 | 20.25 | 51.43 | 109.95 |
| 20.50 | 52.07 | 75.87 | 34.50 | 87.63 | 45.27 | 20.50 | 52.07 | 111.31 |
| 20.75 | 52.70 | 76.80 | 34.75 | 88.26 | 45.60 | 20.75 | 52.70 | 112.67 |
| 21.00 | 53.34 | 77.72 | 35.00 | 88.90 | 45.93 | 21.00 | 53.34 | 114.02 |
| 21.25 | 53.97 | 78.65 | 35.25 | 89.53 | 46.25 | 21.25 | 53.97 | 115.38 |
| 21.50 | 54.61 | 79.57 | 35.50 | 90.17 | 46.58 | 21.50 | 54.61 | 116.74 |
| 21.75 | 55.24 | 80.50 | 35.75 | 90.80 | 46.91 | 21.75 | 55.24 | 118.10 |
| 22.00 | 55.88 | 81.42 | 36.00 | 91.44 | 47.24 | 22.00 | 55.88 | 119.45 |
| | | | 36.25 | 92.07 | 47.57 | | | |
| | | | 36.50 | 92.71 | 47.89 | | | |
| | | | 36.75 | 93.34 | 48.22 | | | |
| | | | 37.00 | 93.98 | 48.55 | | | |
| | | | 37.25 | 94.61 | 48.88 | | | |
| | | | 37.50 | 95.25 | 49.21 | | | |
| | | | 37.75 | 95.88 | 49.54 | | | |
| | | | 38.00 | 96.52 | 49.86 | | | |
| | | | 38.25 | 97.15 | 50.19 | | | |
| | | | 38.50 | 97.79 | 50.52 | | | |
| | | | 38.75 | 98.42 | 50.85 | | | |
| | | | 39.00 | 99.06 | 51.18 | | | |
| | | | 39.25 | 99.69 | 51.50 | | | |
| | | | 39.50 | 100.33 | 51.83 | | | |
| | | | 39.75 | 100.96 | 52.16 | | | |
| | | | 40.00 | 101.60 | 52.49 | | | |
| | | | 40.25 | 102.23 | 52.82 | | | |
| | | | 40.50 | 102.87 | 53.14 | | | |
| | | | 40.75 | 103.50 | 53.47 | | | |
| | | | 41.00 | 104.14 | 53.80 | | | |
| | | | 41.25 | 104.77 | 54.13 | | | |
| | | | 41.50 | 105.41 | 54.46 | | | |
| | | | 41.75 | 106.04 | 54.78 | | | |
| | | | 42.00 | 106.68 | 55.11 | | | |

Note: Percent Fat = Constant A + Constant B − 10.2
[a]Copyright © 1986, 1991, 1996, 2000 by Frank I. Katch, Victor L. Katch, and William D. McArdle, and Fitness Technologies, Inc., 1132 Lincoln Ave. Ann Arbor, MI, 48104. No part of this appendix may be reproduced in any manner without written permission from the copyright holders.

| TABLE 4-5 | Conversion Constants to Predict Percent Body Fat for Older Men[a] | | | | | | | |
|---|---|---|---|---|---|---|---|---|
| **Buttocks** | | | **Abdomen** | | | **Forearm** | | |
| in | cm | Constant A | in | cm | Constant B | in | cm | Constant C |
| 28.00 | 71.12 | 29.34 | 25.50 | 64.77 | 22.84 | 7.00 | 17.78 | 21.01 |
| 28.25 | 71.75 | 29.60 | 25.75 | 65.40 | 23.06 | 7.25 | 18.41 | 21.76 |
| 28.50 | 72.39 | 29.87 | 26.00 | 66.04 | 23.29 | 7.50 | 19.05 | 22.52 |
| 28.75 | 73.02 | 30.13 | 26.25 | 66.67 | 23.51 | 7.75 | 19.68 | 23.26 |
| 29.00 | 73.66 | 30.39 | 26.50 | 67.31 | 23.73 | 8.00 | 20.32 | 24.02 |
| 29.25 | 74.29 | 30.65 | 26.75 | 67.94 | 23.96 | 8.25 | 20.95 | 24.76 |
| 29.50 | 74.93 | 30.92 | 27.00 | 68.58 | 24.18 | 8.50 | 21.59 | 25.52 |
| 29.75 | 75.56 | 31.18 | 27.25 | 69.21 | 24.40 | 8.75 | 22.22 | 26.26 |
| 30.00 | 76.20 | 31.44 | 27.50 | 69.85 | 24.63 | 9.00 | 22.86 | 27.02 |
| 30.25 | 76.83 | 31.70 | 27.75 | 70.48 | 24.85 | 9.25 | 23.49 | 27.76 |
| 30.50 | 77.47 | 31.96 | 28.00 | 71.12 | 25.08 | 9.50 | 24.13 | 28.52 |
| 30.75 | 78.10 | 32.22 | 28.25 | 71.75 | 25.29 | 9.75 | 24.76 | 29.26 |
| 31.00 | 78.74 | 32.49 | 28.50 | 72.39 | 25.52 | 10.00 | 25.40 | 30.02 |
| 31.25 | 79.37 | 32.75 | 28.75 | 73.02 | 25.75 | 10.25 | 26.03 | 30.76 |
| 31.50 | 80.01 | 33.01 | 29.00 | 73.66 | 25.97 | 10.50 | 26.67 | 31.52 |
| 31.75 | 80.64 | 33.27 | 29.25 | 74.29 | 26.19 | 10.75 | 27.30 | 32.27 |
| 32.00 | 81.28 | 33.54 | 29.50 | 74.93 | 26.42 | 11.00 | 27.94 | 33.02 |
| 32.25 | 81.91 | 33.80 | 29.75 | 75.56 | 26.64 | 11.25 | 28.57 | 33.77 |
| 32.50 | 82.55 | 34.06 | 30.00 | 76.20 | 26.87 | 11.50 | 29.21 | 34.52 |
| 32.75 | 83.18 | 34.32 | 30.25 | 76.83 | 27.09 | 11.75 | 29.84 | 35.27 |
| 33.00 | 83.82 | 34.58 | 30.50 | 77.47 | 27.32 | 12.00 | 30.48 | 36.02 |
| 33.25 | 84.45 | 34.84 | 30.75 | 78.10 | 27.54 | 12.25 | 31.11 | 36.77 |
| 33.50 | 85.09 | 35.11 | 31.00 | 78.74 | 27.76 | 12.50 | 31.75 | 37.53 |
| 33.75 | 85.72 | 35.37 | 31.25 | 79.37 | 27.98 | 12.75 | 32.38 | 38.27 |
| 34.00 | 86.36 | 35.63 | 31.50 | 80.01 | 28.21 | 13.00 | 33.02 | 39.03 |
| 34.25 | 86.99 | 35.89 | 31.75 | 80.64 | 28.43 | 13.25 | 33.65 | 39.77 |
| 34.50 | 87.63 | 36.16 | 32.00 | 81.28 | 28.66 | 13.50 | 34.29 | 40.53 |
| 34.75 | 88.26 | 36.42 | 32.25 | 81.91 | 28.88 | 13.75 | 34.92 | 41.27 |
| 35.00 | 88.90 | 36.68 | 32.50 | 82.55 | 29.11 | 14.00 | 35.56 | 42.03 |
| 35.25 | 89.53 | 36.94 | 32.75 | 83.18 | 29.33 | 14.25 | 36.19 | 42.77 |
| 35.50 | 90.17 | 37.20 | 33.00 | 83.82 | 29.55 | 14.50 | 36.83 | 43.53 |
| 35.75 | 90.80 | 37.46 | 33.25 | 84.45 | 29.78 | 14.75 | 37.46 | 44.27 |
| 36.00 | 91.44 | 37.73 | 33.50 | 85.09 | 30.00 | 15.00 | 38.10 | 45.03 |
| 36.25 | 92.07 | 37.99 | 33.75 | 85.72 | 30.22 | 15.25 | 38.73 | 45.77 |
| 36.50 | 92.71 | 38.25 | 34.00 | 86.36 | 30.45 | 15.50 | 39.37 | 46.53 |
| 36.75 | 93.34 | 38.51 | 34.25 | 86.99 | 30.67 | 15.75 | 40.00 | 47.28 |
| 37.00 | 93.98 | 38.78 | 34.50 | 87.63 | 30.89 | 16.00 | 40.64 | 48.03 |
| 37.25 | 94.61 | 39.04 | 34.75 | 88.26 | 31.12 | 16.25 | 41.27 | 48.78 |
| 37.50 | 95.25 | 39.30 | 35.00 | 88.90 | 31.35 | 16.50 | 41.91 | 49.53 |
| 37.75 | 95.88 | 39.56 | 35.25 | 89.53 | 31.57 | 16.75 | 42.54 | 50.28 |
| 38.00 | 96.52 | 39.82 | 35.50 | 90.17 | 31.79 | 17.00 | 43.18 | 51.03 |
| 38.25 | 97.15 | 40.08 | 35.75 | 90.80 | 32.02 | 17.25 | 43.81 | 51.78 |
| 38.50 | 97.79 | 40.35 | 36.00 | 91.44 | 32.24 | 17.50 | 44.45 | 52.54 |
| 38.75 | 98.42 | 40.61 | 36.25 | 92.07 | 32.46 | 17.75 | 45.08 | 53.28 |

*(continued)*

| TABLE 4-5 | CONVERSION CONSTANTS TO PREDICT PERCENT BODY FAT FOR OLDER MEN[a] *(Continued)* | | | | | | | |
|---|---|---|---|---|---|---|---|---|
| **Buttocks** | | | **Abdomen** | | | **Forearm** | | |
| in | cm | Constant A | in | cm | Constant B | in | cm | Constant C |
| 39.00 | 99.06 | 40.87 | 36.50 | 92.71 | 32.69 | 18.00 | 45.72 | 54.04 |
| 39.25 | 99.69 | 41.13 | 36.75 | 93.34 | 32.91 | 18.25 | 46.35 | 54.78 |
| 39.50 | 100.33 | 41.39 | 37.00 | 93.98 | 33.14 | | | |
| 39.75 | 100.96 | 41.66 | 37.25 | 94.61 | 33.36 | | | |
| 40.00 | 101.60 | 41.92 | 37.50 | 95.25 | 33.58 | | | |
| 40.25 | 102.23 | 42.18 | 37.75 | 95.88 | 33.81 | | | |
| 40.50 | 102.87 | 42.44 | 38.00 | 96.52 | 34.03 | | | |
| 40.75 | 103.50 | 42.70 | 38.25 | 97.15 | 34.26 | | | |
| 41.00 | 104.14 | 42.97 | 38.50 | 97.79 | 34.48 | | | |
| 41.25 | 104.77 | 43.23 | 38.75 | 98.42 | 34.70 | | | |
| 41.50 | 105.41 | 43.49 | 39.00 | 99.06 | 34.93 | | | |
| 41.75 | 106.04 | 43.75 | 39.25 | 99.69 | 35.15 | | | |
| 42.00 | 106.68 | 44.02 | 39.50 | 100.33 | 35.38 | | | |
| 42.25 | 107.31 | 44.28 | 39.75 | 100.96 | 35.59 | | | |
| 42.50 | 107.95 | 44.54 | 40.00 | 101.60 | 35.82 | | | |
| 42.75 | 108.58 | 44.80 | 40.25 | 102.23 | 36.05 | | | |
| 43.00 | 109.22 | 45.06 | 40.50 | 102.87 | 36.27 | | | |
| 43.25 | 109.85 | 45.32 | 40.75 | 103.50 | 36.49 | | | |
| 43.50 | 110.49 | 45.59 | 41.00 | 104.14 | 36.72 | | | |
| 43.75 | 111.12 | 45.85 | 41.25 | 104.77 | 36.94 | | | |
| 44.00 | 111.76 | 46.12 | 41.50 | 105.41 | 37.17 | | | |
| 44.25 | 112.39 | 46.37 | 41.75 | 106.04 | 37.39 | | | |
| 44.50 | 113.03 | 46.64 | 42.00 | 106.68 | 37.62 | | | |
| 44.75 | 113.66 | 46.89 | 42.25 | 107.31 | 37.87 | | | |
| 45.00 | 114.30 | 47.16 | 42.50 | 107.95 | 38.06 | | | |
| 45.25 | 114.93 | 47.42 | 42.75 | 108.58 | 38.28 | | | |
| 45.50 | 115.57 | 47.68 | 43.00 | 109.22 | 38.51 | | | |
| 45.75 | 116.20 | 47.94 | 43.25 | 109.85 | 38.73 | | | |
| 46.00 | 116.84 | 48.21 | 43.50 | 110.49 | 38.96 | | | |
| 46.25 | 117.47 | 48.47 | 43.75 | 111.12 | 39.18 | | | |
| 46.50 | 118.11 | 48.73 | 44.00 | 111.76 | 39.41 | | | |
| 46.75 | 118.74 | 48.99 | 44.25 | 112.39 | 39.63 | | | |
| 47.00 | 119.38 | 49.26 | 44.50 | 113.03 | 39.85 | | | |
| 47.25 | 120.01 | 49.52 | 44.75 | 113.66 | 40.08 | | | |
| 47.50 | 120.65 | 49.78 | 45.00 | 114.30 | 40.30 | | | |
| 47.75 | 121.28 | 50.04 | | | | | | |
| 48.00 | 121.92 | 50.30 | | | | | | |
| 48.25 | 122.55 | 50.56 | | | | | | |
| 48.50 | 123.19 | 50.83 | | | | | | |
| 48.75 | 123.82 | 51.09 | | | | | | |
| 49.00 | 124.46 | 51.35 | | | | | | |

Note: Percent Fat = Constant A + Constant B − Constant C − 15.0

| TABLE 4-5 | CONVERSION CONSTANTS TO PREDICT PERCENT BODY FAT FOR YOUNG WOMEN[a] | | | | | | | |
|---|---|---|---|---|---|---|---|---|
| **Abdomen** | | | **Thigh** | | | **Forearm** | | |
| in | cm | Constant A | in | cm | Constant B | in | cm | Constant C |
| 20.00 | 50.80 | 26.74 | 14.00 | 35.56 | 29.13 | 6.00 | 15.24 | 25.86 |
| 20.25 | 51.43 | 27.07 | 14.25 | 36.19 | 29.65 | 6.25 | 15.87 | 26.94 |
| 20.50 | 52.07 | 27.41 | 14.50 | 36.83 | 30.17 | 6.50 | 16.51 | 28.02 |
| 20.75 | 52.70 | 27.74 | 14.75 | 37.46 | 30.69 | 6.75 | 17.14 | 29.10 |
| 21.00 | 53.34 | 28.07 | 15.00 | 38.10 | 31.21 | 7.00 | 17.78 | 30.17 |
| 21.25 | 53.97 | 28.41 | 15.25 | 38.73 | 31.73 | 7.25 | 18.41 | 31.25 |
| 21.50 | 54.61 | 28.74 | 15.50 | 39.37 | 32.25 | 7.50 | 19.05 | 32.33 |
| 21.75 | 55.24 | 29.08 | 15.75 | 40.00 | 32.77 | 7.75 | 19.68 | 33.41 |
| 22.00 | 55.88 | 29.41 | 16.00 | 40.64 | 33.29 | 8.00 | 20.32 | 34.48 |
| 22.25 | 56.51 | 29.74 | 16.25 | 41.27 | 33.81 | 8.25 | 20.95 | 35.56 |
| 22.50 | 57.15 | 30.08 | 16.50 | 41.91 | 34.33 | 8.50 | 21.59 | 36.64 |
| 22.75 | 57.78 | 30.41 | 16.75 | 42.54 | 34.85 | 8.75 | 22.22 | 37.72 |
| 23.00 | 58.42 | 30.75 | 17.00 | 43.18 | 35.37 | 9.00 | 22.86 | 38.79 |
| 23.25 | 59.05 | 31.08 | 17.25 | 43.81 | 35.89 | 9.25 | 23.49 | 39.87 |
| 23.50 | 59.69 | 31.42 | 17.50 | 44.45 | 36.41 | 9.50 | 24.13 | 40.95 |
| 23.75 | 60.32 | 31.75 | 17.75 | 45.08 | 36.93 | 9.75 | 24.76 | 42.03 |
| 24.00 | 60.96 | 32.08 | 18.00 | 45.72 | 37.45 | 10.00 | 25.40 | 43.10 |
| 24.25 | 61.59 | 32.42 | 18.25 | 46.35 | 37.97 | 10.25 | 26.03 | 44.18 |
| 24.50 | 62.23 | 32.75 | 18.50 | 46.99 | 38.49 | 10.50 | 26.67 | 45.26 |
| 24.75 | 62.86 | 33.09 | 18.75 | 47.62 | 39.01 | 10.75 | 27.30 | 46.34 |
| 25.00 | 63.50 | 33.42 | 19.00 | 48.26 | 39.53 | 11.00 | 27.94 | 47.41 |
| 25.25 | 64.13 | 33.76 | 19.25 | 48.89 | 40.05 | 11.25 | 28.57 | 48.49 |
| 25.50 | 64.77 | 34.09 | 19.50 | 49.53 | 40.57 | 11.50 | 29.21 | 49.57 |
| 25.75 | 65.40 | 34.42 | 19.75 | 50.16 | 41.09 | 11.75 | 29.84 | 50.65 |
| 26.00 | 66.04 | 34.76 | 20.00 | 50.80 | 41.61 | 12.00 | 30.48 | 51.73 |
| 26.25 | 66.67 | 35.09 | 20.25 | 51.43 | 42.13 | 12.25 | 31.11 | 52.80 |
| 26.50 | 67.31 | 35.43 | 20.50 | 52.07 | 42.65 | 12.50 | 31.75 | 53.88 |
| 26.75 | 67.94 | 35.76 | 20.75 | 52.70 | 43.17 | 12.75 | 32.38 | 54.96 |
| 27.00 | 68.58 | 36.10 | 21.00 | 53.34 | 43.69 | 13.00 | 33.02 | 56.04 |
| 27.25 | 69.21 | 36.43 | 21.25 | 53.97 | 44.21 | 13.25 | 33.65 | 57.11 |
| 27.50 | 69.85 | 36.76 | 21.50 | 54.61 | 44.73 | 13.50 | 34.29 | 58.19 |
| 27.75 | 70.48 | 37.10 | 21.75 | 55.24 | 45.25 | 13.75 | 34.92 | 59.27 |
| 28.00 | 71.12 | 37.43 | 22.00 | 55.88 | 45.77 | 14.00 | 35.56 | 60.35 |
| 28.25 | 71.75 | 37.77 | 22.25 | 56.51 | 46.29 | 14.25 | 36.19 | 61.42 |
| 28.50 | 72.39 | 38.10 | 22.50 | 57.15 | 46.81 | 14.50 | 36.83 | 62.50 |
| 28.75 | 73.02 | 38.43 | 22.75 | 57.78 | 47.33 | 14.75 | 37.46 | 63.58 |
| 29.00 | 73.66 | 38.77 | 23.00 | 58.42 | 47.85 | 15.00 | 38.10 | 64.66 |
| 29.25 | 74.29 | 39.10 | 23.25 | 59.05 | 48.37 | 15.25 | 38.73 | 65.73 |
| 29.50 | 74.93 | 39.44 | 23.50 | 59.69 | 48.89 | 15.50 | 39.37 | 66.81 |
| 29.75 | 75.56 | 39.77 | 23.75 | 60.32 | 49.41 | 15.75 | 40.00 | 67.89 |
| 30.00 | 76.20 | 40.11 | 24.00 | 60.96 | 49.93 | 16.00 | 40.64 | 68.97 |
| 30.25 | 76.83 | 40.44 | 24.25 | 61.59 | 50.45 | 16.25 | 41.27 | 70.04 |
| 30.50 | 77.47 | 40.77 | 24.50 | 62.23 | 50.97 | 16.50 | 41.91 | 71.12 |
| 30.75 | 78.10 | 41.11 | 24.75 | 62.86 | 51.49 | 16.75 | 42.54 | 72.20 |

*(continued)*

## TABLE 4-5   CONVERSION CONSTANTS TO PREDICT PERCENT BODY FAT FOR YOUNG WOMEN[a] *(Continued)*

| Abdomen | | | Thigh | | | Forearm | | |
|---|---|---|---|---|---|---|---|---|
| in | cm | Constant A | in | cm | Constant B | in | cm | Constant C |
| 31.00 | 78.74 | 41.44 | 25.00 | 63.50 | 52.01 | 17.00 | 43.18 | 73.28 |
| 31.25 | 79.37 | 41.78 | 25.25 | 64.13 | 52.53 | 17.25 | 43.81 | 74.36 |
| 31.50 | 80.01 | 42.11 | 25.50 | 64.77 | 53.05 | 17.50 | 44.45 | 75.43 |
| 31.75 | 80.64 | 42.45 | 25.75 | 65.40 | 53.57 | 17.75 | 45.08 | 76.51 |
| 32.00 | 81.28 | 42.78 | 26.00 | 66.04 | 54.09 | 18.00 | 45.72 | 77.59 |
| 32.25 | 81.91 | 43.11 | 26.25 | 66.67 | 54.61 | 18.25 | 46.35 | 78.67 |
| 32.50 | 82.55 | 43.45 | 26.50 | 67.31 | 55.13 | 18.50 | 46.99 | 79.74 |
| 32.75 | 83.18 | 43.78 | 26.75 | 67.94 | 55.65 | 18.75 | 47.62 | 80.82 |
| 33.00 | 83.82 | 44.12 | 27.00 | 68.58 | 56.17 | 19.00 | 48.26 | 81.90 |
| 33.25 | 84.45 | 44.45 | 27.25 | 69.21 | 56.69 | 19.25 | 48.89 | 82.98 |
| 33.50 | 85.09 | 44.78 | 27.50 | 69.85 | 57.21 | 19.50 | 49.53 | 84.05 |
| 33.75 | 85.72 | 45.12 | 27.75 | 70.48 | 57.73 | 19.75 | 50.16 | 85.13 |
| 34.00 | 86.36 | 45.45 | 28.00 | 71.12 | 58.26 | 20.00 | 50.80 | 86.21 |
| 34.25 | 86.99 | 45.79 | 28.25 | 71.75 | 58.78 | | | |
| 34.50 | 87.63 | 46.12 | 28.50 | 72.39 | 59.30 | | | |
| 34.75 | 88.26 | 46.46 | 38.75 | 73.02 | 59.82 | | | |
| 35.00 | 88.90 | 46.79 | 29.00 | 73.66 | 60.34 | | | |
| 35.25 | 89.53 | 47.12 | 29.25 | 74.29 | 60.86 | | | |
| 35.50 | 90.17 | 47.46 | 29.50 | 74.93 | 61.38 | | | |
| 35.75 | 90.80 | 47.79 | 29.75 | 75.56 | 61.90 | | | |
| 36.00 | 91.44 | 48.13 | 30.00 | 76.20 | 62.42 | | | |
| 36.25 | 92.07 | 48.46 | 30.25 | 76.83 | 62.94 | | | |
| 36.50 | 92.71 | 48.80 | 30.50 | 77.47 | 63.46 | | | |
| 36.75 | 93.34 | 49.13 | 30.75 | 78.10 | 63.98 | | | |
| 37.00 | 93.98 | 49.46 | 31.00 | 78.74 | 64.50 | | | |
| 37.25 | 94.61 | 49.80 | 31.25 | 79.37 | 65.02 | | | |
| 37.50 | 95.25 | 50.13 | 31.50 | 80.01 | 65.54 | | | |
| 37.75 | 95.88 | 50.47 | 31.75 | 80.64 | 66.06 | | | |
| 38.00 | 96.52 | 50.80 | 32.00 | 81.28 | 66.58 | | | |
| 38.25 | 97.15 | 51.13 | 32.25 | 81.91 | 67.10 | | | |
| 38.50 | 97.79 | 51.47 | 32.50 | 82.55 | 67.62 | | | |
| 38.75 | 98.42 | 51.80 | 32.75 | 83.18 | 68.14 | | | |
| 39.00 | 99.06 | 52.14 | 33.00 | 83.82 | 68.66 | | | |
| 39.25 | 99.69 | 52.47 | 33.25 | 84.45 | 69.18 | | | |
| 39.50 | 100.33 | 52.81 | 33.50 | 85.09 | 69.70 | | | |
| 39.75 | 100.96 | 53.14 | 33.75 | 85.72 | 70.22 | | | |
| 40.00 | 101.60 | 53.47 | 34.00 | 86.36 | 70.74 | | | |

Note: Percent Fat = Constant A + Constant B − Constant C − 19.6

| TABLE 4-5 | CONVERSION CONSTANTS TO PREDICT PERCENT BODY FAT FOR OLDER WOMEN[a] | | | | | | | |
|---|---|---|---|---|---|---|---|---|
| **Abdomen** | | | **Thigh** | | | **Forearm** | | |
| in | cm | Constant A | in | cm | Constant B | in | cm | Constant C |
| 25.00 | 63.50 | 29.69 | 14.00 | 35.56 | 17.31 | 10.00 | 25.40 | 14.46 |
| 25.25 | 64.13 | 29.98 | 14.25 | 36.19 | 17.62 | 10.25 | 26.03 | 14.82 |
| 25.50 | 64.77 | 30.28 | 14.50 | 36.83 | 17.93 | 10.50 | 26.67 | 15.18 |
| 25.75 | 65.40 | 30.58 | 14.75 | 37.46 | 18.24 | 10.75 | 27.30 | 15.54 |
| 26.00 | 66.04 | 30.87 | 15.00 | 38.10 | 18.55 | 11.00 | 27.94 | 15.91 |
| 26.25 | 66.67 | 31.17 | 15.25 | 38.73 | 18.86 | 11.25 | 28.57 | 16.27 |
| 26.50 | 67.31 | 31.47 | 15.50 | 39.37 | 19.17 | 11.50 | 29.21 | 16.63 |
| 26.75 | 67.94 | 31.76 | 15.75 | 40.00 | 19.47 | 11.75 | 29.84 | 16.99 |
| 27.00 | 68.58 | 32.06 | 16.00 | 40.64 | 19.78 | 12.00 | 30.48 | 17.35 |
| 27.25 | 69.21 | 32.36 | 16.25 | 41.27 | 20.09 | 12.25 | 31.11 | 17.71 |
| 27.50 | 69.85 | 32.65 | 16.50 | 41.91 | 20.40 | 12.50 | 31.75 | 18.08 |
| 27.75 | 70.48 | 32.95 | 16.75 | 42.54 | 20.71 | 12.75 | 32.38 | 18.44 |
| 28.00 | 71.12 | 33.25 | 17.00 | 43.18 | 21.02 | 13.00 | 33.02 | 18.80 |
| 28.25 | 71.75 | 33.55 | 17.25 | 43.81 | 21.33 | 13.25 | 33.65 | 19.16 |
| 28.50 | 72.39 | 33.84 | 17.50 | 44.45 | 21.64 | 13.50 | 34.29 | 19.52 |
| 28.75 | 73.02 | 34.14 | 17.75 | 45.08 | 21.95 | 13.75 | 34.92 | 19.88 |
| 29.00 | 73.66 | 34.44 | 18.00 | 45.72 | 22.26 | 14.00 | 35.56 | 20.24 |
| 29.25 | 74.29 | 34.73 | 18.25 | 46.35 | 22.57 | 14.25 | 36.19 | 20.61 |
| 29.50 | 74.93 | 35.03 | 18.50 | 46.99 | 22.87 | 14.50 | 36.83 | 20.97 |
| 29.75 | 75.56 | 35.33 | 18.75 | 47.62 | 23.18 | 14.75 | 37.46 | 21.33 |
| 30.00 | 76.20 | 35.62 | 19.00 | 38.26 | 23.49 | 15.00 | 38.10 | 21.69 |
| 30.25 | 76.83 | 35.92 | 19.25 | 48.89 | 23.80 | 15.25 | 38.73 | 22.05 |
| 30.50 | 77.47 | 36.22 | 19.50 | 49.53 | 24.11 | 15.50 | 39.37 | 22.41 |
| 30.75 | 78.10 | 36.51 | 19.75 | 50.16 | 24.42 | 15.75 | 40.00 | 22.77 |
| 31.00 | 78.74 | 36.81 | 20.00 | 50.80 | 24.73 | 16.00 | 40.64 | 23.14 |
| 31.25 | 79.37 | 37.11 | 20.25 | 51.43 | 25.04 | 16.25 | 41.27 | 23.50 |
| 31.50 | 80.01 | 37.40 | 20.50 | 52.07 | 25.35 | 16.50 | 41.91 | 23.86 |
| 31.75 | 80.64 | 37.70 | 20.75 | 52.70 | 25.66 | 16.75 | 42.54 | 24.22 |
| 32.00 | 81.28 | 38.00 | 21.00 | 53.34 | 25.97 | 17.00 | 43.18 | 24.58 |
| 32.25 | 81.91 | 38.30 | 21.25 | 53.97 | 26.28 | 17.25 | 43.81 | 24.94 |
| 32.50 | 82.55 | 38.59 | 21.50 | 54.61 | 26.58 | 17.50 | 44.45 | 25.31 |
| 32.75 | 83.18 | 38.89 | 21.75 | 55.24 | 26.89 | 17.75 | 45.08 | 25.67 |
| 33.00 | 83.82 | 39.19 | 22.00 | 55.88 | 27.20 | 18.00 | 45.72 | 26.03 |
| 33.25 | 84.45 | 39.48 | 22.25 | 56.51 | 27.51 | 18.25 | 46.35 | 26.39 |
| 33.50 | 85.09 | 39.78 | 22.50 | 57.15 | 27.82 | 18.50 | 46.99 | 26.75 |
| 33.75 | 85.72 | 40.08 | 22.75 | 57.78 | 28.13 | 18.75 | 47.62 | 27.11 |
| 34.00 | 86.36 | 40.37 | 23.00 | 58.42 | 28.44 | 19.00 | 48.26 | 27.47 |
| 34.25 | 86.99 | 40.67 | 23.25 | 59.05 | 28.75 | 19.25 | 48.89 | 27.84 |
| 34.50 | 87.63 | 40.97 | 23.50 | 59.69 | 29.06 | 19.50 | 49.53 | 28.20 |
| 34.75 | 88.26 | 41.26 | 23.75 | 60.32 | 29.37 | 19.75 | 50.16 | 28.56 |
| 35.00 | 88.90 | 41.56 | 24.00 | 60.96 | 29.68 | 20.00 | 50.80 | 28.92 |
| 35.25 | 89.53 | 41.86 | 24.25 | 61.59 | 29.98 | 20.25 | 51.43 | 29.28 |
| 35.50 | 90.17 | 42.15 | 24.50 | 62.23 | 30.29 | 20.50 | 52.07 | 29.64 |
| 35.75 | 90.80 | 42.45 | 24.75 | 62.86 | 30.60 | 20.75 | 52.70 | 30.00 |

*(continued)*

| TABLE 4-5 | CONVERSION CONSTANTS TO PREDICT PERCENT BODY FAT FOR OLDER WOMEN[a] *(Continued)* | | | | | | | |
|---|---|---|---|---|---|---|---|---|
| | Abdomen | | | Thigh | | | Forearm | |
| in | cm | Constant A | in | cm | Constant B | in | cm | Constant C |
| 36.00 | 91.44 | 42.75 | 25.00 | 63.50 | 30.91 | 21.00 | 53.34 | 30.37 |
| 36.25 | 92.07 | 43.05 | 25.25 | 64.13 | 31.22 | 21.25 | 53.97 | 30.73 |
| 36.50 | 92.71 | 43.34 | 25.50 | 64.77 | 31.53 | 21.50 | 54.61 | 31.09 |
| 36.75 | 93.35 | 43.64 | 25.75 | 65.40 | 31.84 | 21.75 | 55.24 | 31.45 |
| 37.00 | 93.98 | 43.94 | 26.00 | 66.04 | 32.15 | 22.00 | 55.88 | 31.81 |
| 37.25 | 94.62 | 44.23 | 26.25 | 66.67 | 32.46 | 22.25 | 56.51 | 32.17 |
| 37.50 | 95.25 | 44.53 | 26.50 | 67.31 | 32.77 | 22.50 | 57.15 | 32.54 |
| 37.75 | 95.89 | 44.83 | 26.75 | 67.94 | 33.08 | 22.75 | 57.78 | 32.90 |
| 38.00 | 96.52 | 45.12 | 27.00 | 68.58 | 33.38 | 23.00 | 58.42 | 33.26 |
| 38.25 | 97.16 | 45.42 | 27.25 | 69.21 | 33.69 | 23.25 | 59.05 | 33.62 |
| 38.50 | 97.79 | 45.72 | 27.50 | 69.85 | 34.00 | 23.50 | 59.69 | 33.98 |
| 38.75 | 98.43 | 46.01 | 27.75 | 70.48 | 34.31 | 23.75 | 60.32 | 34.34 |
| 39.00 | 99.06 | 46.31 | 28.00 | 71.12 | 34.62 | 24.00 | 60.96 | 34.70 |
| 39.25 | 99.70 | 46.61 | 28.25 | 71.75 | 34.93 | 24.25 | 61.59 | 35.07 |
| 39.50 | 100.33 | 46.90 | 28.50 | 72.39 | 35.24 | 24.50 | 62.23 | 35.43 |
| 39.75 | 100.97 | 47.20 | 28.75 | 73.02 | 35.55 | 24.75 | 62.86 | 35.79 |
| 40.00 | 101.60 | 47.50 | 29.00 | 73.66 | 35.86 | 25.00 | 63.50 | 36.15 |
| 40.25 | 101.24 | 47.79 | 29.25 | 74.29 | 36.17 | | | |
| 40.50 | 102.87 | 48.09 | 29.50 | 74.93 | 36.48 | | | |
| 40.75 | 103.51 | 48.39 | 29.75 | 75.56 | 36.79 | | | |
| 41.00 | 104.14 | 48.69 | 30.00 | 76.20 | 37.09 | | | |
| 41.25 | 104.78 | 48.98 | 30.25 | 76.83 | 37.40 | | | |
| 41.50 | 105.41 | 49.28 | 30.50 | 77.47 | 37.71 | | | |
| 41.75 | 106.05 | 49.58 | 30.75 | 78.10 | 38.02 | | | |
| 42.00 | 106.68 | 49.87 | 31.00 | 78.74 | 38.33 | | | |
| 42.25 | 107.32 | 50.17 | 31.25 | 79.37 | 38.64 | | | |
| 42.50 | 107.95 | 50.47 | 31.50 | 80.01 | 38.95 | | | |
| 42.75 | 108.59 | 50.76 | 31.75 | 80.64 | 39.26 | | | |
| 43.00 | 109.22 | 51.06 | 32.00 | 81.28 | 39.57 | | | |
| 43.25 | 109.86 | 51.36 | 32.25 | 81.91 | 39.88 | | | |
| 43.50 | 110.49 | 51.65 | 32.50 | 82.55 | 40.19 | | | |
| 43.75 | 111.13 | 51.95 | 32.75 | 83.18 | 40.49 | | | |
| 44.00 | 111.76 | 52.25 | 33.00 | 83.82 | 40.80 | | | |
| 44.25 | 112.40 | 52.54 | 33.25 | 84.45 | 41.11 | | | |
| 44.50 | 113.03 | 52.84 | 33.50 | 85.09 | 41.42 | | | |
| 44.75 | 113.67 | 53.14 | 33.75 | 85.72 | 41.73 | | | |
| 45.00 | 114.30 | 53.44 | 34.00 | 86.36 | 42.04 | | | |

Note: Percent Fat = Constant A + Constant B − Constant C − 19.6

| BOX 4-1 | **Standardized Description of Skinfold Sites and Procedures** |
|---------|---------------------------------------------------------------|

*Skinfold Site*

- Abdominal — Vertical fold; 2 cm to the right side of the umbilicus
- Triceps — Vertical fold; on the posterior midline of the upper arm, halfway between the acromion and olecranon processes, with the arm held freely to the side of the body
- Biceps — Vertical fold; on the anterior aspect of the arm over the belly of the biceps muscle, 1 cm above the level used to mark the triceps site
- Chest/Pectoral — Diagonal fold; one-half the distance between the anterior axillary line and the nipple (men) or one-third of the distance between the anterior axillary line and the nipple (women)
- Medial Calf — Vertical fold; at the maximum circumference of the calf on the midline of its medial border
- Midaxillary — Vertical fold; on the midaxillary line at the level of the xiphoid process of the sternum (An alternate method is a horizontal fold taken at the level of the xiphoid/sternal border in the midaxillary line.)
- Subscapular — Diagonal fold (at a 45° angle); 1 to 2 cm below the inferior angle of the scapula
- Suprailiac — Diagonal fold; in line with the natural angle of the iliac crest taken in the anterior axillary. line immediately superior or the iliac crest
- Thigh — Vertical fold; on the anterior midline of the thigh, midway between the proximal border of the patella and the inguinal crease (hip)

*Procedures*

- All measurements should be made on the right side of the body
- Caliper should be placed 1 cm away from the thumb and finger, perpendicular to the skinfold; and halfway between the crest and the base of the fold
- Pinch should be maintained while reading the caliper
- Wait 1 to 2 s (and not longer) before reading caliper
- Take duplicate measures at each site and retest if duplicate measurements are not within 1 to 2 mm
- Rotate through measurement sites or allow time for skin to regain normal texture and thickness

above the site by 1 cm. Place the caliper tips on the double-fold of skin and fat. Note: both right- and left-handed calipers are available.

4. Release the scissor grip of the caliper claws and continue to support the weight of the caliper with that hand.

5. Record the reading on the caliper scale 1 to 2 seconds (and not longer) after releasing the scissor grip lever to allow the jaws of the caliper to measure the skinfold site.

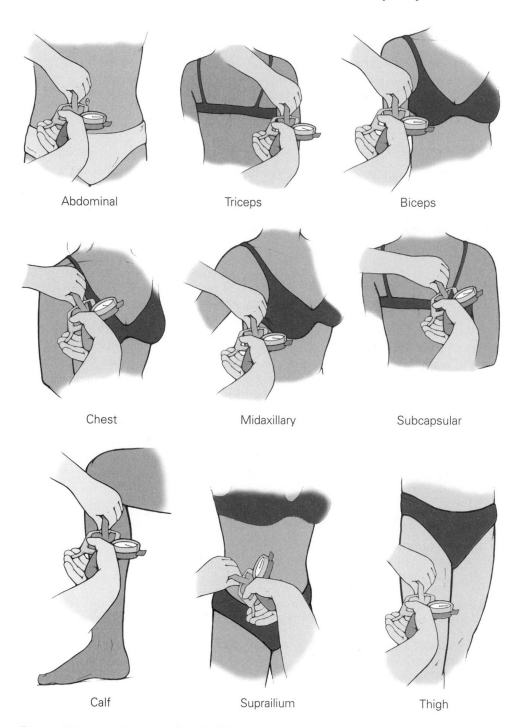

FIGURE 4-8. Anatomical sites for skinfold measurement.

Measure the skinfold to the nearest 0.5 mm (using the Lange caliper). If not within 1 or 2 mm, then retest this site. Be careful to avoid jaw slippage.

6. Measure each skinfold site at least two times. Rotate through the measurement sites to allow time for the skin to regain its normal texture and thickness.

7. Sum the mean, or average, of each skinfold site to determine percent body fat with the specific skinfold formula.

### Equation Selection

To select the most appropriate equation, it is important to consider the following:

- To whom or what special population is the equation applicable?
- Was the appropriate reference method used to develop the equation?
- Was a representative sample of that population studied?
- How were the variables measured?

### Skinfold Prediction Equations

#### JACKSON-POLLOCK 7-SITE SKINFOLD FORMULA FOR BODY DENSITY

Provide averages for the skinfold measurement for the subscapular, triceps, chest, axillary, suprailium, abdominal, and thigh sites. Use these sums in the gender-specific formulas below. The square of the sum of the 7 skinfold sites and the person's age will be also used in the calculation. An example of this calculation can be found below. Note, there are no tables available to determine percent body fat from the sum of these seven skinfold sites; the mathematical formula must be used. This formula solves for body density (BD); BD may then be converted to percent body fat, as shown below using either the Siri or Brozek equations. The 3-site skinfold equations have tables available to help solve for percent body fat. Box 4–2 provides generalized skinfold equations. Percent body fat: can be determined from either the Siri or Brozek equations using BD.

- Siri Equation

$$\% \text{ Body Fat} = \frac{495}{\text{BD}} - 450$$

- Brozek Equation

$$\% \text{ Body Fat} = \frac{457}{\text{BD}} - 414.2$$

These equations are similar in their result, i.e., percent body fat. Lohman (1984) suggested an alternative formula of [% Body Fat = 509 / BD − 465] for young women.

For example: Jackson & Pollock 7 site calculation
Gender = male
Age = 32 years
Means for skinfold sites (in mm):

| | |
|---|---|
| Triceps | 7 |
| Midaxillary | 11 |
| Chest | 9 |
| Subscapular | 12 |
| Suprailium | 13 |
| Abdominal | 15 |
| Thigh | 15 |

Sum of 7 sites = 82 mm
$\text{Sum}^2 = 6724$

Male formula:

BD = 1.112 − 0.00043499 (82) + 0.00000055 (6724) − 0.00028826 (32)

You can use scientific notation (EE) on the calculator to solve (scientific notation in parentheses), or you may have to round off numbers to fit into the calculator's memory.

First multiply each factor out (scientific notation in parentheses):

0.00043499 (4.3499 EE − .04) · 82 =  0.035669 (3.5669 EE − 02)
0.00000055 (5.5 EE −.07) · 6724  =  0.0036982 (3.6982 EE − 03)
0.00028826 (2.8826 EE −.04) · 32  =  0.0092243 (9.2243 EE − 03)

Then put all values back into equation:

BD  = 1.112 − (3.5669 EE − 02) + (3.6982 EE − 03) − (9.2243 EE − 03)
    = 1.0708

% Body Fat = $\frac{495 − 450}{BD}$ (Siri equation)

= $\frac{495 − 450}{1.0708}$

= 12.27%

(using the Brozek equation, % Body Fat = 12.78%)

---

**BOX 4-2    Generalized Skinfold Equations***

*Men*
- **7-Site Formula** (chest, midaxillary, triceps, subscapular, abdomen, suprailiac, thigh)
  Body Density = 1.112 − 0.00043499 (Sum of 7 Skinfolds) + 0.00000055 (Sum of 7 Skinfolds)$^2$ − 0.00028826 (Age)
- **3-Site Formula** (chest, abdomen, thigh)
  Body Density = 1.10938 − 0.0008267 (Sum of 3 Skinfolds) + 0.0000016 (Sum of 3 Skinfolds)$^2$ − 0.0002574 (Age)
- **3-Site Formula** (chest, triceps, subscapular)
  Body Density = 1.1125025 − 0.0013125 (Sum of 3 Skinfolds) + 0.0000055 (Sum of 3 Skinfolds)$^2$ − 0.000244 (Age)

*Women*
- **7-Site Formula** (chest, midaxillary, triceps, subscapular, abdomen, suprailiac, thigh)
  Body Density = 1.097 − 0.00046971 (Sum of 7 Skinfolds) + 0.00000056 (Sum of 7 Skinfolds)$^2$ − 0.00012828 (Age)
- **3-Site Formula** (triceps, suprailiac, thigh)
  Body Density = 1.099421 − 0.0009929 (Sum of 3 Skinfolds) + 0.0000023 (Sum of 3 Skinfolds)$^2$ − 0.0001392 (Age)
- **3-Site Formula** (triceps, suprailiac, abdominal)
  Body Density = 1.089733 − 0.0009245 (Sum of 3 Skinfolds) + 0.0000025 (Sum of 3 Skinfolds)$^2$ − 0.0000979 (Age)

*Adapted from Jackson AS, Pollock ML. Practical assessment of body comparison. Physician Sport Med 1985:13:76–90.

JACKSON-POLLOCK 3-SITE SKINFOLD FORMULAS FOR BODY DENSITY

Skinfold sites:

| J-P 3-site (1980) | J-P 3-site (1985) |
|---|---|
| Women: | Women: |
| Triceps | Triceps |
| Suprailiac | Suprailiac |
| Thigh | Abdominal |
| Men: | Men: |
| Chest | Chest |
| Thigh | Triceps |
| Abdominal | Subscapular |

## Bioelectrical Impedance Analysis

Bioelectrical impedance analysis (BIA) is a non-invasive and easy to administer method for assessing body composition. The basic premise behind the procedure is that the volume of fat-free tissue in the body will be proportional to the electrical conductivity of the body. Thus, the bioelectrical impedance analyzer passes a small electrical current into the body and then measures the resistance to that current. The theory behind BIA is that fat is a poor electrical conductor containing little water (14–22%), while lean tissue contains mostly water (more than 90%) and electrolytes and is a good electrical conductor. Thus, fat tissue is an impedance to electrical current. In actuality, BIA measures total body water and uses calculations for percent body fat using some assumptions about hydration levels of individuals and the exact water content of various tissues. The following conditions must be controlled to ensure the subject has a normal hydration level so the BIA measurement is valid.

- No eating or drinking within 4 hours of the test.
- No exercise within 12 hours of the test.
- Urinate (or void) completely within 30 minutes of the test.
- No alcohol consumption in the previous 48 hours before the test.
- No diuretics in the 7 days before the test (unless prescribed by a physician).
- Limited use of diuretic agents (i.e., caffeine, chocolate, etc.) before the test.

### Procedures for BIA

1. Calibrate the BIA machine according to manufacturer's instructions.
2. Prepare the subject for the test by having them lie down on the table. Have the subject remove all jewelry. The subject will need to remove the right sock and shoe.
3. Do not allow the subject's legs or arms to touch each other.
4. Wipe the right ankle/foot and right wrist/hand sites with an alcohol pad.
5. Place the four electrodes on the body anatomically:
   - Right wrist: midpoint on line bisecting ulna and radius styloid processes.
   - Right hand: on distal metacarpal (knuckle of index finger).
   - Right ankle: midpoint on line bisecting medial and lateral malleoli.
   - Right foot: on distal metatarsal (knuckle of big toe).
     The red electrode attachments go to the proximal electrodes—wrist and ankle (red = close to heart). The black electrode attachments go to the distal electrodes—hand and foot.
6. Follow the specific analyzer's procedures for computer input information and test collection.

## Hydrostatic Weighing

Underwater weighing (UWW) is considered a criterion, or gold standard, method for body composition analysis. This method uses Archimedes' principle that the density of the body is equal to the mass of the body divided by its volume. The density of the body can then be converted to percent body fat using either the previously presented Siri or Brozek equations. All other methods of body composition analyses (e.g., skinfolds, BIA, etc.) are based on, or depend on, UWW. Thus, all other methods can only be as accurate as UWW. In this technique (also known as densitometry), the body is divided into two components: fat mass (FM) and fat-free mass (FFM). This separation into only two components has been questioned by some experts stating there are more than two components in the human body that need to be considered for body composition analysis.

For the UWW method, several variables must be known:

- Residual volume: the amount of air remaining in the lungs after full expiration; this air will aid in buoyancy, potentially increasing the percent body fat.
- Density of the water: the density of the water varies with its temperature. Buoyancy will decrease with warmer water temperatures.
- Trapped gas in gastrointestinal system: a constant of 100 mL is used for all trapped gas in the gastrointestinal system; this gas will also aid buoyancy.
- Body weight in air (dry).
- Body weight fully submerged in water (wet).

Next, the density of the body may be calculated and converted to percent body fat by using either the Siri or Brozek equations.

### Procedures for UWW

1. Subject should wear a bathing suit (nylon is best). The suit should not add to buoyancy by trapping air.
2. The subject should be relatively clean of body oils and should have urinated and defecated, if possible, before the procedure.
3. The subject should remove all jewelry.
4. Normal hydration of the subject is desirable. Women should not be tested within 7 days on either side of menstruation. The subject should be 3 to 12 hours post-absorptive.
5. The body of water for UWW should be as small and controlled as possible. The temperature should be between 33 to 36°C (91–97°F). The water should be chlorinated. The density of the water should be determined based on its temperature (this measurement can be found in many different textbooks, ranging from chemistry to exercise physiology).
6. First, weigh the subject (in kilograms) dry (on land) and with as little clothing on as is practical. Convert this weight from kilograms to grams (multiply by 1000).
7. Calculate, or predict, their residual volume (RV) based upon their height (cm) and age:
   - Male RV (L): $[0.019 \cdot HT \text{ (cm)}] + [0.0155 \cdot \text{age (yrs)}] - 2.24$
   - Female RV (L): $[0.032 \cdot HT \text{ (cm)}] + [0.009 \cdot \text{age (yrs)}] - 3.90$
8. Convert this RV from Liters to milliliters (multiply by 1000). Note: the RV can also be measured by various pulmonary function tests; however, this measurement is relatively sophisticated or difficult to make. The actual measurement of RV greatly increases the accuracy of the UWW method.
9. Weigh the individual underwater several times (5–10). Each weighing should be done after a deep, full expiration. The subject needs to be fully submerged and at residual

volume. The subject may have to stay submerged for 5 to 10 seconds. The movement of the subject in the chair (or apparatus) should be minimal to decrease the fluctuations on the weight scale. Oftentimes a cadaver scale or vegetable scale is used to weigh submerged people; however, a force-transducer system is more accurate.

10. Often the greatest weight of the subject is used for the UWW or perhaps an averaging of the two or three highest weights.

11. The density of the body may be determined from the equation below. Then percent body fat can be calculated using Table 4-6.

**TABLE 4-6** POPULATION-SPECIFIC FORMULAS FOR CONVERSION OF BODY DENSITY (DB) TO PERCENT BODY FAT*

| Population | Age | Gender | % Body Fat† |
|---|---|---|---|
| **Race** | | | |
| *American Indian* | 18–60 | Female | (4.81/Db)-4.34 |
| *Black* | 18–32 | Male | (4.37/Db)-3.93 |
| | 24–79 | Female | (4.85/Db)-4.39 |
| *Hispanic* | 20–40 | Female | (4.87/Db)-4.41 |
| *Japanese Native* | 18–48 | Male | (4.97/Db)-4.52 |
| | | Female | (4.76/Db)-4.28 |
| | 61–78 | Male | (4.87/Db)-4.41 |
| | | Female | (4.95/Db)-4.50 |
| *White* | 7–12 | Male | (5.30/Db)-4.89 |
| | | Female | (5.35/Db)-4.95 |
| | 13–16 | Male | (5.07/Db)-4.64 |
| | | Female | (5.10/Db)-4.66 |
| | 17–19 | Male | (4.99/Db)-4.55 |
| | | Female | (5.05/Db)-4.62 |
| | 20–80 | Male | (4.95/Db)-4.50 |
| | | Female | (5.01/Db)-4.57 |
| **Levels of Body Fatness** | | | |
| *Anorexia* | 15–30 | Female | (5.26/Db)-4.83 |
| *Obese* | 17–62 | Male | (5.00/Db)-4.56 |

Adapted from Heyward VH, Stolarczyk LM. Applied Body Comparison Assessment Champaign, IL: Human Kinetics, 1996.
†Percent body fat is obtained by multiplying the value calculated from the equation by 100.

## Formula for UWW

$$BD = \frac{WT \text{ in air (gm)}}{\left[ \dfrac{WT \text{ in air (gm)} - WT \text{ in water (gm)}}{Density \text{ of water}} \right] - [RV \text{ (mL)}]}$$

Note: BD is likely to be between 1.020–1.090.

- Siri equation: % Body Fat $= \dfrac{495}{BD} - 450$

- Brozek equation: % Body Fat $= \dfrac{457}{BD} - 414.2$

For example:

Male: WT = 83.62 kg or 83,620 gm
HT = 172 cm; Age = 27 years
RV predicted = 1.338 L or 1,338 mL
Water Temperature = 32°C
Density of water = 0.9950 (@ 32°C)
UWW = 4.37 kg or 4370 g

$$BD = \frac{83,620}{\dfrac{[83,620 - 4,370] - [1,338]}{0.9950}}$$

$$BD = \frac{83,620}{79,648 - 1,338}$$

$$BD = \frac{83,620}{78,310}$$

$$BD = 1.0678$$

$$\% \text{ Body Fat} = \frac{495 - 450 \text{ (Siri)}}{1.0678}$$

$$\% \text{ Body Fat} = 13.6\%$$

## SUMMARY OF BODY COMPOSITION METHODOLOGY

Height/Weight Tables:
• Subjective
• May be based on a limited sample of clients who sought out life insurance
• Problem with the definition of frame size (visual or elbow breadth)
• Problem with the definition of overweight versus overfat

Body Mass Index (BMI):
• Simple calculation of the ratio of height to weight (similar concerns as Height/Weight Tables)
• Popular with large scale (epidemiological) studies
• Good morbidity and mortality statistics available

Waist-to-Hip Ratio (WHR):
• Simple measure to obtain
• Ratio is not interpretable by itself
• The association of WHR to morbidity and mortality is impressive and perhaps causal
• Can use waist circumference alone

Circumferences (girths):
• Many formulas for converting to percent body fat
• Problem of girth size not directly related to fat
• Fairly simple yet not as accurate as skinfolds
• May be a good method for demonstrating body composition, or size, changes over time

Skinfolds:
• Highly regarded technique, yet prone to error
• Technician training important

- Anatomical site selection crucial
- Many skinfold formulas exist from one site up to 10 sites and some formulas that combine with some circumference measures
- Not more accurate than underwater weighing, privacy issue

Bioelectrical Impedance Analysis (BIA):
- Newer technique that attempts to eliminate technician error
- Dependent on many assumptions that client must meet (e.g., body water or hydration level)
- No more accurate than skinfolds and more costly; probably quicker than skinfolds and less privacy required

Underwater Weighing (hydrostatic or densitometry):
- Time consuming
- Costly in equipment and technicians, training
- Equipment size
- Reference standard
- Clients may be less likely to prefer this method
- Issue of extra effort to perform procedure versus increase in accuracy

## Calculation of Ideal or Desired Body Weight

Along with the determination of percent body fat, it is often desirable to determine an ideal or desired body weight based on a desired percent body fat for the individual. Obviously, this process can be problematic in that a desirable percent body fat for an individual must be determined. The determination of a desirable body weight is useful in weight loss or maintenance.

$$\text{Ideal Body Weight (IBW) Calculations} = \frac{\text{LBM (Lean Body Mass)}}{1.00 - (\text{Desired \% Body Fat}/100)}$$

For example:
If a man weighs 190 lbs and is measured to have 22.3% body fat, then:

Fat Weight
$= \text{Body Weight} \cdot (\text{\% Body Fat}/100)$
$= 190 \cdot (22.3/100)$
$= 42.37 \text{ lbs}$

Lean Body Mass (LBM)
(Fat Free Weight)
$= \text{Body Weight} - \text{Fat Weight}$
$= 190 - 42.37$
$= 147.63 \text{ lbs}$

Ideal Body Weight (IBW)
$= \dfrac{147.63}{1.00 - (15/100)}$
(15% used for a man as a guideline)
$= 173.68 \ (@ \ 15\% \text{ body fat})$

Weight Loss
$= \text{Body Weight} - \text{Ideal Body Weight}$

In this example, $190 - 173.7 = 16.3$ lbs of weight to lose to achieve ideal body weight.

## Simple Weight Management: Application of Calorie Determination

Obesity is the surplus of fat stored resulting from excess energy intake relative to energy expenditure. Exercise is a key component to weight management:

- Exercise expends energy
- Exercise may suppress appetite
- Exercise can minimize the loss of lean body mass
- Exercise can counter the impact on resting metabolic rate (RMR) from dieting
  Energy Balance Theory = Calories IN (Food Intake) − Calories OUT (Activity)

This is an oversimplified area: open to much misunderstanding by both the public and professionals. It states that if a client eats more calories than they expend, they would gain weight. And, if one expends more calories than they eat, they would lose weight. This theory or equation comes from a simple law in physics that energy can neither be created nor destroyed. Unfortunately, this energy balance theory or equation does not seem to work exactly in humans and weight maintenance (loss or gain).

One simplification of weight loss is 1 lb of FAT = 3500 calories. This can be useful with dietary factors and exercise when discussing weight management (e.g., 2 cookies is about 115 kcals; 30 days of 2 extra cookies per day = 1 lb weight gain). If you walk 1 mile (or run 1 mile), then you use approximately 100 kcal. If you walk 1 mile per day for a year, then you should lose 10.5 lbs. You can apply the ACSM Metabolic Calculation Equations for energy expenditure for different modes of exercise (i.e., walking, etc.) to determine the caloric expenditure and relate this to ideal weight and weight management.

## LABORATORY EXERCISES

1. Measure the body composition of at least one individual, using several different methods (i.e., BMI, WHR, BIA, skinfolds, underwater weighing, etc.). Compare and contrast the calculations of the various measures using the data sheet provided.

*Suggested Readings*

1. ACSM's Guidelines for Exercise Testing and Prescription, 6th ed. Baltimore: Lippincott Williams & Wilkins, 2000.
2. ACSM's Resource Manual for Guidelines for Exercise Testing and Prescription. 4th ed. Baltimore: Lippincott Williams & Wilkins, 2001.
3. Heyward VH, Stolarczyk LM. Applied Body Composition Assessment. Champaign, IL: Human Kinetics, 1996.
4. Lohman TG. Advances in Body Composition Assessment. Champaign, IL: Human Kinetics, 1992.
5. Lohman TG, Roche AF, Martorell R. Anthropometric Standardization Reference Manual. Champaign, IL: Human Kinetics, 1988.

# 5

# Muscular Fitness:
## *Muscular Strength, Muscular Endurance, and Flexibility*

Experts in the field of physical fitness have included "muscular fitness" as a component of health-related physical fitness, along with cardiorespiratory fitness, body composition, and flexibility. Muscular fitness is a 'linked' term that integrates muscular strength and muscular endurance. Thus, the term muscular fitness has been derived to infer this inter-dependence. Flexibility refers to the ability to move a joint through its complete range of motion. Consequently, maintaining flexibility of all joints facilitates movement. Therefore, the importance of these three components to achieve enhanced health-related physical fitness is apparent.

Development and maintenance of muscular fitness contributes to:

- Increasing fat-free mass and resting metabolic rate
- Maintaining bone mass
- Modest improvements in cardiovascular fitness
- Improved ability to perform activities of daily living (ADLs)

## DEFINING MUSCULAR STRENGTH

The definition of muscular strength is the maximal force that can be generated by a specific muscle or muscle group. Muscle strength is specific to the muscle group, type of contraction (static or dynamic; concentric or eccentric), the speed of the contraction, and the joint angle being tested. Therefore, no single assessment exists for evaluating total body muscular strength. The measurement of muscle force production is used for the following:

- To assess muscular fitness
- To identify weaknesses
- To monitor progress in rehabilitation
- To measure effectiveness of training

## DEFINING MUSCULAR ENDURANCE

The definition of muscular endurance is the ability of a muscle group to execute repeated contractions over a period of time sufficient to cause muscular fatigue, or to maintain a specific percentage of the maximum voluntary contraction for a prolonged period of time.

The testing of muscular strength and muscular endurance, the two components of health-related physical fitness, is far from standardized. Experts disagree with the test modes used to assess or evaluate these components. Before describing specific assessment tools, the following should be considered:

- Participants should be familiarized with the equipment and procedures.
- Equipment should be reviewed for safety.
- The participant should be encouraged to exhale during concentric contraction and inhale during eccentric contraction.
- Adequate rest should be provided between assessments.

## COMMON ASSESSMENTS FOR MUSCULAR STRENGTH
### Handgrip Test
*Procedures*

1. The subject should be standing for the test. One procedure for this test is to have the subject perform the test with each hand. The norms listed below use a combined score for the right and left hands. Another procedure, not discussed here, is to have the subject use their dominant hand.

2. Adjust the grip bar to fit comfortably within the subject's hand. The second joint of the fingers should 'fit' under the handle of the handgrip dynamometer. Make sure that the handgrip dynamometer is set back to zero.
3. Have the subject hold the handgrip dynamometer parallel to the side of the body at about waist level. The forearm should be level with the thigh. The subject may flex the arm slightly.
4. The subject should then squeeze the handgrip dynamometer as hard as possible with care not to hold their breath (Valsalva maneuver).
5. Record the grip strength in kilograms. Repeat this procedure using the opposite hand.
6. Repeat the test two more times with each hand. Take the highest of the three readings for each hand and add these two values (one from each hand) together as the measure of handgrip strength to compare to the norms presented in Table 5-1.

## Norms for Grip Strength (Table 5-1)

| TABLE 5-1 | GRIP-STRENGTH (KG) NORMS BY AGE GROUPS AND GENDER FOR COMBINED RIGHT AND LEFT HAND | | | | | |
|---|---|---|---|---|---|---|
| Age (yrs) | 15–19 | | 20–29 | | 30–39 | |
| Gender | M | F | M | F | M | F |
| Above average | 103–112 | 64–70 | 113–123 | 65–70 | 113–122 | 66–72 |
| Average | 95–102 | 59–63 | 106–112 | 61–64 | 105–112 | 61–65 |
| Below average | 84–94 | 54–58 | 97–105 | 55–60 | 97–104 | 56–60 |
| Poor | ≤83 | ≤53 | ≤96 | ≤54 | ≤96 | ≤55 |

| Age (yrs) | 40–49 | | 50–59 | | 60–69 | |
|---|---|---|---|---|---|---|
| Gender | M | F | M | F | M | F |
| Above average | 110–118 | 65–72 | 102–109 | 59–64 | 98–101 | 54–59 |
| Average | 102–109 | 59–64 | 96–101 | 55–58 | 86–92 | 51–53 |
| Below average | 94–101 | 55–58 | 87–95 | 51–54 | 79–85 | 48–50 |
| Poor | ≤93 | ≤54 | ≤86 | ≤50 | ≤78 | ≤47 |

Adapted from *The Canadian Physical Activity, Fitness & Lifestyle Appraisal: CSEP's Plan for Healthy Active Living*, 1996. Reprinted by permission from the Canadian Society for Exercise Physiology.

## 1-REPETITION MAXIMUM (RM) BENCH PRESS TEST

Definition: 1-RM stands for a one time maximum amount of weight lifted. Research has shown that the single best weight lifting test for predicting total dynamic strength is the 1-RM bench press. The test measures the strength of the muscles involved in arm extension; triceps, pectoralis major, and anterior deltoid. This test can be time consuming and complicated to perform to determine a subject's absolute maximum amount of weight that can be lifted.

## Procedures

1. Allow the subject to become comfortable with the bench press and its operation by practicing a light warm-up of 5 to 10 repetitions at 40 to 60% of perceived maximum.

2. For the test, the subject is to keep the back on the bench, both feet on the floor, and the hands should be shoulder width apart with palms up on the bar. Free-weight equipment is preferred over equipment like Universal or Nautilus. A spotter must be present for all lifts. The spotter hands the bar to the subject. The subject starts the lift with the bar in the up position and arms fully extended. The bar is lowered to the chest and then pushed back up until the arms are locked. Be mindful of breathing; avoid a Valsalva maneuver (holding breath).

3. Following a 1-minute rest with light stretching, the subject does 3 to 5 repetitions at 60 to 80% of perceived maximum.

4. The subject should be close to the perceived maximum. Add a small amount of weight and a 1-RM lift is attempted. If the lift is successful, then a rest period of 3 to 5 minutes is provided. The goal is to find the 1-RM in 3 to 5 maximal efforts. The process continues until a failed attempt occurs. The greatest amount of weight lifted is considered the 1-RM.

5. For a ratio determination of the amount of weight lifted compared to the individual's body weight (for norms comparison purposes), divide the maximum weight lifted in pounds by the subject's weight in pounds.

Note: The above procedure can be used for the 1-RM leg press.

## Norms for Upper Body Strength (Table 5-2)

| TABLE 5-2 | UPPER BODY STRENGTH*,† | | | | |
|---|---|---|---|---|---|
| | Age | | | | |
| Percentile | 20–29 | 30–39 | 40–49 | 50–59 | 60+ |
| *Men* | | | | | |
| 90 | 1.48 | 1.24 | 1.10 | .97 | .89 |
| 80 | 1.32 | 1.12 | 1.00 | .90 | .82 |
| 70 | 1.22 | 1.04 | .93 | .84 | .77 |
| 60 | 1.14 | .98 | .88 | .79 | .72 |
| 50 | 1.06 | .93 | .84 | .75 | .68 |
| 40 | .99 | .88 | .80 | .71 | .66 |
| 30 | .93 | .83 | .76 | .68 | .63 |
| 20 | .88 | .78 | .72 | .63 | .57 |
| 10 | .80 | .71 | .65 | .57 | .53 |
| *Women* | | | | | |
| 90 | .90 | .76 | .71 | .61 | .64 |
| 80 | .80 | .70 | .62 | .55 | .54 |
| 70 | .74 | .63 | .57 | .52 | .51 |
| 60 | .70 | .60 | .54 | .48 | .47 |
| 50 | .65 | .57 | .52 | .46 | .45 |
| 40 | .59 | .53 | .50 | .44 | .43 |
| 30 | .56 | .51 | .47 | .42 | .40 |
| 20 | .51 | .47 | .43 | .39 | .38 |
| 10 | .48 | .42 | .38 | .37 | .33 |

*One repetition maximum bench press, with bench press weight ratio = weight pushed/body weight ratio.
† Data provided by the Institute for Aerobics Research, Dallas, TX (1994). Adapted from ACSM's *Guidelines for Exercise Testing and Prescription* 6th ed. Study population for the data set was predominantly white and college educated. A Universal dynamic variable resistance (DVR) machine was used to measure the I-RM. The following may be used as descriptors for the percentile rankings: well above average (90), above average (70), average (50); below average (30), and well below average (10).

## Norms for Leg Strength (Table 5-3)

| TABLE 5-3 | LEG STRENGTH*,† | | | | |
|---|---|---|---|---|---|
| | **Age** | | | | |
| **Percentile** | **20–29** | **30–39** | **40–49** | **50–59** | **60+** |
| *Men* | | | | | |
| 90 | 2.27 | 2.07 | 1.92 | 1.80 | 1.73 |
| 80 | 2.13 | 1.93 | 1.82 | 1.71 | 1.62 |
| 70 | 2.05 | 1.85 | 1.74 | 1.64 | 1.56 |
| 60 | 1.97 | 1.77 | 1.68 | 1.58 | 1.49 |
| 50 | 1.91 | 1.71 | 1.62 | 1.52 | 1.43 |
| 40 | 1.83 | 1.65 | 1.57 | 1.46 | 1.38 |
| 30 | 1.74 | 1.59 | 1.51 | 1.39 | 1.30 |
| 20 | 1.63 | 1.52 | 1.44 | 1.32 | 1.25 |
| 10 | 1.51 | 1.43 | 1.35 | 1.22 | 1.16 |
| *Women* | | | | | |
| 90 | 1.82 | 1.61 | 1.48 | 1.37 | 1.32 |
| 80 | 1.68 | 1.47 | 1.37 | 1.25 | 1.18 |
| 70 | 1.58 | 1.39 | 1.29 | 1.17 | 1.13 |
| 60 | 1.50 | 1.33 | 1.23 | 1.10 | 1.04 |
| 50 | 1.44 | 1.27 | 1.18 | 1.05 | .99 |
| 40 | 1.37 | 1.21 | 1.13 | .99 | .93 |
| 30 | 1.27 | 1.15 | 1.08 | .95 | .88 |
| 20 | 1.22 | 1.09 | 1.02 | .88 | .85 |
| 10 | 1.14 | 1.00 | .94 | .78 | .72 |

*One repetition maximum leg press with leg press weight ratio = weight pushed body weight.
† Data provided by the Institute for Aerobics Research, Dallas, TX (1994). Adapted from *ACSM's Guidelines for Exercise Testing and Prescription,* 6th ed. Study population for the data set was predominantly white and college educated. A Universal dynamic variable resistance (DVR) machine was used to measure the I-RM. The following may be used as descriptors for the percentile rankings: well above average (90), above average (70), average (50); below average (30), and well below average (10).

## Isokinetic Testing

This involves constant-speed muscular contraction against accommodating resistance. The speed of movement is controlled and the amount of resistance is proportional to the amount of force produced throughout the full range of motion. A variety of commercial devices are available that will measure peak force and torque of various joints (knee, hip, shoulder, elbow). The drawback is the expense of the equipment.

## COMMON ASSESSMENTS FOR MUSCULAR ENDURANCE

### Partial Curl-Up and Push-Up Tests

*Procedures (Box 5-1)*

*Norms for Partial Curl-Up (Table 5-4)*

*Position for Partial Curl-Up (Fig. 5-1)*

*Norms for Push-Ups (Table 5-5)*

| BOX 5-1 | Push-Up and Curl-Up (Crunch) Test Procedures for Measurement of Muscular Endurance |
|---|---|

*Push-Up*
1. The push-up test is administered with male subjects in the standard "up" position (hands shoulder width apart, back straight, head up, using the toes as the pivotal point) and female subjects in the modified "knee push-up" position (legs together, lower leg in contact with mat with ankles plantar-flexed, back straight, hands shoulder width apart, head up).
2. The subject must lower the body until the chin touches the mat. The stomach should not touch the mat (41).
3. For both men and women, the subject's back must be straight at all times and the subject must push up to a straight arm position.
4. The maximal number of push-ups performed consecutively without rest is counted as the score.

*Curl-Up (Crunch)*
1. Individual assumes a supine position on a mat with the knees at 90°. The arms are at the side, with fingers touching a piece of masking tape. A second piece of masking tape is placed 8 cm (for those who are ≥45 v) or 12 cm (for those who are <45 v) beyond the first (40).*
2. A metronome is set to 40 beats · min¹ and the individual does slow, controlled curl-ups to hit the shoulder blades off the mat (trunk males a 30° angle with the mat) in time with the metronome (20 curl-ups/min). The low back should be flattened before curling up.
3. Individual performs as many curl-ups as possible without pausing, up to a maximum of 75.

*Alternatives include (a) having the hands held across the chest, with the head activating a counter when the trunk reaches a 30° position (39) and placing the hands on the thighs and curling up until the hands reach the knee caps (40). Elevation of the trunk to 30° is the important aspect of the movement.

† An alternative includes doing as many curl-ups as possible in 1 minute (39).

| TABLE 5-4 | PERCENTILES BY AGE GROUPS AND GENDER FOR PARTIAL CURL-UP* |
|---|---|

| | Age | | | | | | | | | |
|---|---|---|---|---|---|---|---|---|---|---|
| Percentile | 20–29 | | 30–39 | | 40–49 | | 50–59 | | 60–69 | |
| Gender | M | F | M | F | M | F | M | F | M | F |
| 90 | 75 | 70 | 75 | 55 | 75 | 50 | 74 | 48 | 53 | 50 |
| 80 | 56 | 45 | 69 | 43 | 75 | 42 | 60 | 30 | 33 | 30 |
| 70 | 41 | 37 | 46 | 34 | 67 | 33 | 45 | 23 | 26 | 24 |
| 60 | 31 | 32 | 36 | 28 | 51 | 28 | 35 | 16 | 19 | 19 |
| 50 | 27 | 27 | 31 | 21 | 39 | 25 | 27 | 9 | 16 | 13 |
| 40 | 24 | 21 | 26 | 15 | 31 | 20 | 23 | 2 | 9 | 9 |
| 30 | 20 | 17 | 19 | 12 | 26 | 14 | 19 | 0 | 6 | 3 |
| 20 | 13 | 12 | 13 | 0 | 21 | 5 | 13 | 0 | 0 | 0 |
| 10 | 4 | 5 | 0 | 0 | 13 | 0 | 0 | 0 | 0 | 0 |

*Based on data from Canadian Standardized Test of Fitness Operations Manual 3rd ed. Ottawa: Canadian Society for Exercise Physiology in cooperation with Fitness Canada, Government of Canada, 1986. The following may be used as descriptors for the percentile rankings: well above average (90), above average (70), average (50), below average (30), and well below average (10).

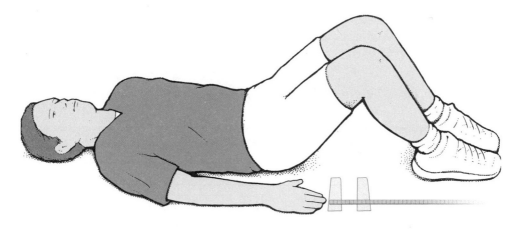

**FIGURE 5-1.** Partial curl-up.

## YMCA Bench Press Test

*Procedures*

1. Use a 35-pound barbell setup for women or an 80-pound barbell setup for men.
2. Set the metronome to 60 beats per minute, the subject's lifting cadence will be 30 lifts or reps per minute.
3. Have the subject lie back down on the bench with both feet on the floor.
4. A spotter should hand the barbell to the subject and be available throughout the test to grasp the barbell when necessary.
5. The subject will start with the weight in the down position (weight resting on chest) and with elbows flexed. Hands should grip the bar at shoulder width with palms up.
6. The subject will press the weight up and lower the weight at the cadence of 30 repetitions per minute. Each repetition must consist of full movement of the barbell from elbows flexed with the barbell resting on the chest to arms fully extended. The cadence of 30 repetitions per minute must be maintained.

| TABLE 5-5 | PERCENTILES BY AGE GROUPS AND GENDER FOR PUSH-UPS* | | | | | | | | | |
|---|---|---|---|---|---|---|---|---|---|---|
| | **Age** | | | | | | | | | |
| **Percentile** | **20–29** | | **30–39** | | **40–49** | | **50–59** | | **60–69** | |
| **Gender** | **M** | **F** | **M** | **F** | **M** | **F** | **M** | **F** | **M** | **F** |
| 90 | 41 | 32 | 32 | 31 | 25 | 28 | 24 | 23 | 24 | 25 |
| 80 | 34 | 26 | 27 | 24 | 21 | 22 | 17 | 17 | 16 | 15 |
| 70 | 30 | 22 | 24 | 21 | 19 | 18 | 14 | 13 | 11 | 12 |
| 60 | 27 | 20 | 21 | 17 | 16 | 14 | 11 | 10 | 10 | 10 |
| 50 | 24 | 16 | 19 | 14 | 13 | 12 | 10 | 9 | 9 | 6 |
| 40 | 21 | 14 | 16 | 12 | 12 | 10 | 9 | 5 | 7 | 4 |
| 30 | 18 | 11 | 14 | 10 | 10 | 7 | 7 | 3 | 6 | 2 |
| 20 | 16 | 9 | 11 | 7 | 8 | 4 | 5 | 1 | 4 | — |
| 10 | 11 | 5 | 8 | 4 | 5 | 2 | 4 | — | 2 | — |

*Based on data from the Canada Fitness Survey, 1981. (Reprinted from Canadian Standardized Test of Fittness (CSTF) Operations Manual. 3rd ed. With permission of Fitness Canada, Fitness and Amateur Sport Canada, Ottawa, 1986.) The following may be used as descriptors for the percentile rankings: well above average (90), above average (70), average (50), below average (30), and well below average (10).

7. The subject completes the test for the maximum number of repetitions before fatigue or breaking of the lifting cadence. Compare the subject's maximum number of reps to the norms (Table 5-6).

## Norms for YMCA Bench Press (Table 5-6)

| TABLE 5-6 | ENDURANCE BENCH-PRESS TEST—TOTAL LIFTS | | | | | |
|---|---|---|---|---|---|---|
| Age (yrs) | 18–25 | | 26–35 | | 36–45 | |
| Gender | M | F | M | F | M | F |
| Excellent | 44–64 | 42–66 | 41–61 | 40–62 | 36–55 | 33–57 |
| Good | 34–41 | 30–38 | 30–37 | 29–34 | 26–32 | 26–30 |
| Above average | 29–33 | 25–28 | 26–29 | 24–28 | 22–25 | 21–24 |
| Average | 24–28 | 20–22 | 21–24 | 18–22 | 18–21 | 16–20 |
| Below average | 20–22 | 16–18 | 17–20 | 14–17 | 14–17 | 12–14 |
| Poor | 13–17 | 9–13 | 12–16 | 9–13 | 9–12 | 6–10 |
| Very poor | 0–10 | 0–6 | 0–9 | 0–6 | 0–6 | 0–4 |

| Age (yrs) | 46–55 | | 56–65 | | >65 | |
|---|---|---|---|---|---|---|
| Gender | M | F | M | F | M | F |
| Excellent | 28–47 | 29–50 | 24–41 | 24–42 | 20–36 | 18–30 |
| Good | 21–25 | 20–24 | 17–21 | 17–21 | 12–16 | 12–16 |
| Above Average | 16–20 | 14–18 | 12–14 | 12–14 | 10 | 8–10 |
| Average | 12–14 | 10–13 | 9–11 | 8–10 | 7–8 | 5–7 |
| Below average | 9–11 | 7–9 | 5–8 | 5–6 | 4–6 | 3–4 |
| Poor | 5–8 | 2–6 | 2–4 | 2–4 | 2–3 | 0–2 |
| Very Poor | 0–2 | 0–1 | 0–1 | 0–1 | 0–1 | 0 |

*Note:* Women use a 35-pound bar; men, 80 pounds. Maximum repetitions in time to metronome at 30 lifts per minute.
*Source:* Adapted from YMCA. *Y'S Way to Fitness,* 4th ed., 1998. Reprinted with permission from the YMCA of the USA.

## DEFINING FLEXIBILITY

Flexibility is the functional capacity of the joints to move through a full range of motion (ROM). The functional ROM refers to the ability to move the joint without incurring pain or a limit to performance. Flexibility depends on which muscle and joint is being evaluated; therefore, it is joint-specific. In addition, flexibility depends on the distensibility of the joint capsule, adequate warm-up, muscle viscosity, and the compliance of ligaments and tendons.

Flexibility assessment is necessary because of the associated decreased performance of activities of daily living with inadequate flexibility. Poor lower back and hip flexibility may contribute to the development of muscular lower back pain.

There is no single test that can truly characterize one's flexibility; however, the sit and reach test is the most widely used test for the assessment of flexibility. It does not represent total body flexibility, but it does represent hamstring, hip, and lower back flexibility.

A variety of assessments of flexibility should be performed to provide the professional with a profile of overall flexibility.

## Sit and Reach Test (Trunk Flexion)

### Procedures (Box 5-2)

1. Before administering the sit and reach test, offer the individual the opportunity to do some stretching exercises and light to moderate aerobic exercise (5–10 minutes) to warm up the muscles. Inquire whether the subject has any back problems before administering the protocol. If the subject has a back problem or has a history of back problems:
2. Make sure that they have an adequate aerobic and muscular warm-up
3. Have them take a few practice tries before the actual measure and inquire if it bothers the back, or skip the test.

---

| BOX 5-2 | **Trunk Flexion (Sit-and-Reach) Test Procedures\*** |
|---|---|

**Pretest:** Participant should perform a short warm-up prior to this test and include some stretches (e.g., modified hurdler's stretch). It is also recommended that the participant refrain from fast, jerky movements, which may increase the possibility of an injury. The participant's shoes should be removed.

1. For the YMCA sit-and-reach test, a yardstick is placed on the floor and tape is placed across it at a right angle to the 15-inch mark. The participant sits with the yardstick between the legs, with legs extended at right angles to the taped line on the floor. Heels of the feet should touch the edge of the taped line and be about 10 to 12 inches apart. If a standard sit-and-reach box is available, heels should be placed against the edge of the box.
2. The participant should slowly reach forward with both hands as far as possible, holding this position momentarily. Be sure that the participant keeps the hands parallel and does not lead with one hand. Fingertips can be overlapped and should be in contact with the yardstick or measuring portion of the sit-and-reach box.
3. The score is the most distant point (in inches or centimeters) reached with the fingertips. The best of three trials should be recorded. To assist with the best attempt, the participant should exhale and drop the head between the arms when reaching. Testers should ensure that the knees of the participant stay extended: however, the participant's knees should not be pressed down. The participant should breathe normally during the test and should not hold his or her breath at any time. Norms for the YMCA test are presented in Table 5-8.
4. The sit-and-reach test is also done using a sit-and-reach box. The participant sits with the legs fully extended with the soles of the feet against the box. The other directions are as described above. Norms for a sit-and-reach box test are provided in Table 4-12. Note that these norms use a sit-and-reach box in which the "zero" point is set at the 26 cm mark (41). If you are using a box in which the zero point is set at 23 cm (e.g., Fitnessgram), subtract 3 cm from each value in this table.

---

\*Diagrams of these procedures are available elsewhere.

*Norms for Sit and Reach Test (Table 5-7)*

*Position for Sit and Reach Test (Fig. 5-2)*

| **TABLE 5-7** | **Percentiles by Age Groups for Trunk Forward Flexion Using a Sit-and-Reach Box (cm)\*** | | | | | | | | | |
|---|---|---|---|---|---|---|---|---|---|---|
| | **Age** | | | | | | | | | |
| **Percentile** | **20–29** | | **30–39** | | **40–49** | | **50–59** | | **60–69** | |
| **Gender** | **M** | **F** | **M** | **F** | **M** | **F** | **M** | **F** | **M** | **F** |
| 90 | 42 | 43 | 40 | 42 | 37 | 40 | 38 | 40 | 35 | 37 |
| 80 | 38 | 40 | 37 | 39 | 34 | 37 | 32 | 37 | 30 | 34 |
| 70 | 36 | 38 | 34 | 37 | 30 | 35 | 29 | 33 | 26 | 31 |
| 60 | 33 | 36 | 32 | 35 | 28 | 33 | 27 | 32 | 24 | 30 |
| 50 | 31 | 34 | 29 | 33 | 25 | 31 | 25 | 30 | 22 | 28 |
| 40 | 29 | 32 | 27 | 31 | 23 | 29 | 22 | 29 | 18 | 26 |
| 30 | 26 | 29 | 24 | 28 | 20 | 26 | 18 | 26 | 16 | 24 |
| 20 | 23 | 26 | 21 | 25 | 16 | 24 | 15 | 23 | 14 | 23 |
| 10 | 18 | 22 | 17 | 21 | 12 | 19 | 12 | 19 | 11 | 18 |

\*Based on data from the Canada fitness survey, 1981. Reprinted from Canadian Standardized Test of Fitness ICSTF Operations Manual, 3rd ed. With permission of Fitness Canada, Fitness and Amateur Sport Canada, Ottawa, 1986. The following may be used as descriptors for the percentile rankings: well above average (90), above average (70), average (70), below average (30), and well below average (10).
Note: these norms are based on a sit-and-reach box in which the "zero" point is set at 26 cm. When using a box in which the "zero" point is set at 23 cm. subtract 3 cm from each value in this table

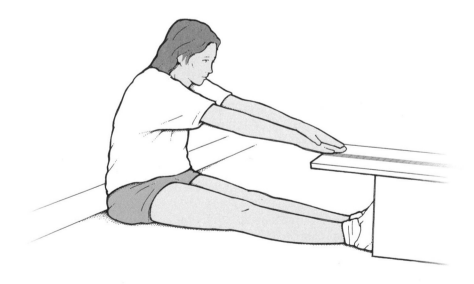

**Figure 5-2.** Sit and reach.

## YMCA Sit and Reach Test

*Procedures (Box 5-2)*

1. To prepare the subject for the YMCA sit and reach test is the same as for the aforementioned protocol.

**TABLE 5-8    PERCENTILES BY AGE GROUPS AND GENDER FOR YMCA SIT-AND-REACH TEST (INCHES)\***

| Percentile | Age | | | | | | | | | | | |
|---|---|---|---|---|---|---|---|---|---|---|---|---|
| | 18–25 | | 26–35 | | 36–45 | | 46–55 | | 56–65 | | >65 | |
| Gender | M | F | M | F | M | F | M | F | M | F | M | F |
| 90 | 22 | 24 | 21 | 23 | 21 | 22 | 19 | 21 | 17 | 20 | 17 | 20 |
| 80 | 20 | 22 | 19 | 21 | 19 | 21 | 17 | 20 | 15 | 19 | 15 | 18 |
| 70 | 19 | 21 | 17 | 20 | 17 | 19 | 15 | 18 | 13 | 17 | 13 | 17 |
| 60 | 18 | 20 | 17 | 20 | 16 | 18 | 14 | 17 | 13 | 16 | 12 | 17 |
| 50 | 17 | 19 | 15 | 19 | 15 | 17 | 13 | 16 | 11 | 15 | 10 | 15 |
| 40 | 15 | 18 | 14 | 17 | 13 | 16 | 11 | 14 | 9 | 14 | 9 | 14 |
| 30 | 14 | 17 | 13 | 16 | 13 | 15 | 10 | 14 | 9 | 13 | 8 | 13 |
| 20 | 13 | 16 | 11 | 15 | 11 | 14 | 9 | 12 | 7 | 11 | 7 | 11 |
| 10 | 11 | 14 | 9 | 13 | – | 12 | 6 | 10 | 5 | 9 | 4 | 9 |

\*Based on data from YMCA of the USA (reference 18). The following may be used as descriptors for the percentile rankings: well above average (90), above average (70), average (50), below average (30), and well below average (10)

2. For the YMCA sit and reach test, a yardstick is placed on the floor and tape is placed across it at a right angle to the 15-inch mark.
3. The subject sits with the yardstick between the legs and the legs extended at right angles to the taped line on the floor. Heels of the feet should touch the edge of the taped line and be about 10 to 12 inches apart.
4. Repeat the remainder of procedures from the previous protocol.

*Norms for YMCA Sit and Reach Test (Table 5-8)*

## RECOMMENDED EQUIPMENT FOR ADDITIONAL TESTS (BOX 5-3)

Other tests for flexibility include the laboratory assessment of the ROM of a specific joint using a goniometer to measure joint movement in degrees. Common devices for this include goniometers, electrogoniometers, the Leighton flexometer, inclinometers, and tape

**BOX 5-3    Recommended Equipment for Additional Tests**

*Muscular Strength*
Free weights (barbells, dumbells)
Variable-resistance machines
Iso-kinetic machines (if available)
Handgrip dynamometer
Flexibility

*Goniometers*
Sit and reach box

*Muscular Endurance*
Free weights (barbells, dumbells)
Gym mat (curl-ups, push-ups)
Stopwatch

measures. The MacRae and Wright (MW) Test is a criterion measure for lower back flexibility, and the straight-leg raise is a criterion measure for hamstring flexibility.

### Procedures for the MacRae-Wright (MW) Back Criterion Test

1. Subject stands erect.
2. Locate the sacroiliac joint by palpation and mark it with a pen.
3. Measure and mark the points 5 cm below and 10 cm above the lumbosacral joint mark (total distance 15 cm).
4. Subject sits with legs extended on the floor, mat, table, or bench.
5. View the marks on the subject's back while placing the tape measure on the low 5 cm mark.
6. As the subject bends maximally forward, measure the distance from the lowest mark to the highest mark.
7. Subtract the original position 15 cm from the maximally stretched position's distance.
8. The procedure is repeated three times, with the average being recorded as the flexibility score.

### Procedures for the Goniometric Hamstring Criterion Test

1. Align the axis of the goniometer with the axis of subject's hip joint.
2. Place the stationary arm of the goniometer in line with the trunk and the mobile arm in line with the femur.
3. Hold the subject's knee straight while moving that leg toward hip flexion.
4. The leg is held while a reading to the closest degree is made from the angle produced by the stationary arm and mobile arm of the goniometer.
5. The average of three trials is used as a flexibility score.

## LABORATORY EXERCISES

1. Select a subject and complete the following assessments. Remember to begin evaluation with an explanation of procedures, warm-up, and safety measures.

   Subject: _____    Gender: _____    Age: _____

   Muscular Strength:
      Handgrip
         Right Hand                              Left Hand
            Trial I _____ kg                    Trial I _____ kg
            Trial II _____ kg                   Trial II _____ kg
            Trial III _____ kg                  Trial III _____ kg
            Max Score$_1$ _____ kg              Max Score$_2$ _____ kg
      Total Score: Max Score$_1$ + Max Score$_2$ = _____    Norms Rating: _____

   Muscular Endurance:
      Curl-ups
         Total Score: _____    Norms Rating: _____
      Push-ups
         Total Score: _____    Norms Rating: _____

Flexibility:

   Sit and reach

      Trial I _____

      Trial II _____        Best Trial: _____

      Trial III _____     Norm Rating: _____

## Suggested Readings

1. ACSM's Guidelines for Exercise Testing and Prescription, 6th ed. Baltimore: Lippincott Williams & Wilkins, 2000.
2. ACSM's Resource Manual for Guidelines for Testing and Exercise Prescription, 4th ed. Baltimore: Lippincott Williams & Wilkins, 2001.
3. American College of Sports Medicine. Position stand: The recommended quantity and quality of exercise for developing and maintaining cardiorespiratory and muscular fitness in healthy adults. Med Sci Sports Exer 1990;22:265–274.
4. Fleck SJ, Kraemer WJ. Designing Resistance Training Programs, 2nd ed. Champaign, IL: Human Kinetics, 1997.

# 6

# Cardiorespiratory Fitness Measurement:

## *Step Tests and Field Tests to Predict Cardiorespiratory Fitness*

Cardiorespiratory fitness (CRF) reflects the functional capabilities of the heart, blood vessels, blood, lungs, and relevant muscles during various types of exercise demands. Specifically, CRF affects numerous physiological responses: at rest, in response to submaximal exercise, in response to maximal exercise, and during prolonged work.

CRF is related to the ability to perform large muscle, dynamic, moderate-to-high intensity exercise for prolonged periods. CRF is a synonym for many terms that may be used for the same thing (e.g., aerobic capacity; see below). This can be confusing. The following is a list of the terms that all mean essentially the same thing:

- Maximal Aerobic Capacity
- Functional Capacity
- Physical Work Capacity (PWC)
- Maximal Oxygen Uptake or Consumption
- $VO_{2max}$ or $VO_{2peak}$
- Cardiovascular *Endurance, Fitness, or Capacity*
- Cardiorespiratory *Endurance, Fitness, or Capacity*
- Cardiopulmonary *Endurance, Fitness, or Capacity*

In this chapter, we will discuss the measurement (by prediction) of CRF by the use of field tests such as the 1.5 mile run test and step tests. In subsequent chapters of this manual, we will explore both submaximal and maximal exercise tests.

## THE CONTINUUM OF MEASUREMENT OF CRF

CRF can be measured or predicted using many methods. There are three general types of assessment tests for CRF discussed in this manual:

- Field Tests: having the subject perform a timed completion of a certain distance, complete a measured distance, or perform for a set time to predict CRF. These tests generally demand maximal effort for the best score in CRF. The testing modes include walk, walk-run, run, cycle, swim, and others.
- Submaximal Exertion: using either step test or a single-stage or a multi-stage submaximal exercise protocol to predict maximal aerobic capacity or CRF from submaximal measures of efficiency of certain measured variables (usually heart rate response). Testing modes include steps, treadmill, cycle, and others. While some may consider step tests to be in part a submaximal exertion test, for the purpose of this manual, step tests will be described in this chapter. Many of these tests will be performed in a laboratory setting.
- Maximal Exertion: using a graded or progressive exercise test to measure an individual's volitional fatigue or exhaustion. Thus, this test is to maximal exertion. This test involves a measure of CRF rather than a prediction. This test may or may not involve the collection of metabolic gases and is likely performed in a laboratory setting.

## IMPORTANCE OF MEASUREMENT OF CRF

The fitness professional needs to decide what test may be the most appropriate for CRF determination for a client. The measurement of CRF can be justified for use in:

- Exercise prescription and programming: in helping to set up an exercise program
- Progress and motivation of an individual in an exercise program: in providing both feedback and motivation to keep a client interested in exercise
- Prediction of medical conditions such as coronary heart disease: in helping to further pick up or diagnose health problems

The true measurement of CRF involves maximal exertion or exercise, along with collection of expired gases. The measurement of expired gases is not always applicable, nor desirable, to many settings that wish to measure or quantify CRF such as corporate fitness and wellness programs. Thus, there are many approaches to the assessment of CRF that do not involve the use of maximal exercise and/or the use of sophisticated gas analyzers.

This area of assessment has the important concept of the prediction of CRF. Most CRF assessment tests, except maximal graded exercise testing with collection of expired gases, use prediction techniques to 'calculate' the maximal oxygen uptake, or $VO_{2max}$. There is always error associated with any prediction test (e.g., submaximal cycle ergometry). Some important questions related to prediction and errors are:

- How important is the prediction error?
- Can you accept this prediction error?
- Can you explain this prediction error to your clients?

Because of the numerous options for assessment tests for CRF, the choice of which test to use is important. Some of the factors that may help the decision of which test to use are:

- Time demands
- Expense or costs
- Personnel needed (i.e., qualifications)
- Equipment and facilities needed
- Physician supervision needed
- Population tested (i.e., safety concerns)
- Need for accuracy of data

## PRE-TEST CONSIDERATIONS

The pre-test considerations for all clients who undergo these various tests for aerobic capacity are important to standardize the testing conditions. This can also increase the accuracy of prediction of CRF and help the client's safety. The instructions to the client before the test can increase the level of comfort as well. These general instructions are:

- Abstain from eating prior (> 4 hours); however, make sure the client has eaten recently to avoid hypoglycemia.
- Abstain from strenuous exercise before (> 24 hours)
- Abstain from caffeine products before (> 12–24 hours)
- Abstain from nicotine products before (> 3 hours)
- Abstain from alcohol before (> 24 hours)
- Medications considerations (if the client's medications affect resting or exercise heart rate (HR), it will invalidate the test)

The use of health screening before any exercise test is important. The ACSM guidelines should be used for risk stratification to help decide about the need for a maximal exercise test before starting an exercise program and to determine if a physician should be present during either a submaximal or maximal exercise test. These guidelines were discussed in Chapter 2.

## STEP TESTS

Step tests have been around for over 50 years in fitness testing. There are many protocols that have been developed that use a step test to predict CRF. We will discuss the use of the McArdle or Queens College Step Test for the prediction of aerobic capacity. This test relies on having the subject step up and down on a standardized step or bench (standardized for step height) for a set period of time at a set stepping cadence. After the test time period is complete, a recovery HR is obtained and used in the prediction of aerobic capacity. The lower the recovery HR, the more fit the individual. Thus, most step tests use the client's HR response to a standard amount of exertion. In general, step tests require little equipment to conduct—perhaps all is needed is a watch, a metronome, and a standardized height step bench. It would be difficult to put a price tag on a bench step because many are home built, as opposed to being from a commercial vendor. Special precautions for safety are needed for those clients who may have balance problems or difficulty with stepping. While step tests may be considered submaximal for many clients, they might be at or near maximal exertion for other clients.

There are several step tests to be found in the literature. This manual will describe the Queen's College Step Test. Other step tests available usually vary from the Queen's College Step Test in either step height and/or test time. Two other popular step tests include the Forestry Test and the Harvard Step Test.

## Queens College Step Test Procedures

The Queens College Step Test is also known as the McArdle Step Test.

1. The step test requires that the individual step up and down on a standardized step height of 16.25 in (41.25 cm) for 3 minutes. (Many gymnasium bleachers have a riser height of 16.25 in.)
2. The men step at a rate (cadence) of 24 per minute, while the women step at a rate of 22 per minute. This cadence should be closely monitored and set with the use of an electronic metronome. A 24 per minute cadence means that the complete cycle of step up with one leg, step up with the other, step down with the first leg, and finally step down with the last leg is performed 24 times in a minute (up one leg, up the other leg, down the first leg, down the other leg). Commonly we set the metronome at a cadence of 4 times the step rate, in this case 96 beats per minute for men, to coordinate each leg's movement with a beat of the metronome. The women's step rate would be 88 beats per minute. While it may be possible to test more than one client at a time, depending on equipment, it would be difficult to test men and women together.
3. After the 3 minutes are up, the client stops and palpates the pulse or has the pulse taken (at the radial site, preferably) while standing within the first 5 seconds. A 15 second pulse count is then taken. Multiply this pulse count by 4 to determine HR in beats per minute (bpm). The recovery HR should occur between 5 and 20 seconds of immediate recovery from the end of the step test.

The Subject's $VO_{2max}$ in $mL \cdot kg^{-1} \cdot min^{-1}$ is determined from the recovery HR by the following formulas:

For Men:
$$VO_{2max} (mL \cdot kg^{-1} \cdot min^{-1}) = 111.33 - (0.42 \cdot HR)$$

For Women:
$$VO_{2max} (mL \cdot kg^{-1} \cdot min^{-1}) = 65.81 - (0.1847 \cdot HR)$$
HR = recovery HR (bpm)

For example:
If a man finished the test with a recovery HR of 144 bpm (36 beats in 15 seconds), then:
$$VO_{2max} (mL \cdot kg^{-1} \cdot min^{-1}) = 111.33 - (0.42 \cdot 144)$$
$$= 50.85 \ mL \cdot kg^{-1} \cdot min^{-1}$$

# FIELD TESTS FOR PREDICTION OF AEROBIC CAPACITY

A field test generally requires the client to perform a task in a non-laboratory to field setting, such as running 1.5 miles at near maximal exertion. For safety reasons, field tests, considered by some to be submaximal, may be inappropriate for sedentary individuals at moderate to high risk for cardiovascular or musculoskeletal complications. There are two common types of tests used for the prediction of aerobic capacity in the field setting: either a timed completion of a set distance (e.g., 1.5-mile run) or a maximal distance for a set time (e.g., 12-minute walk/run). Field tests are relatively easy and inexpensive to administer, therefore, they are ideal for testing large groups of subjects.

## Walk/Run Performance Tests

There are two common field test protocols that use a walk or run performance test to predict aerobic capacity. These walk or run tests tend to be more accurate (less error in prediction) than the step tests discussed in the last section. The performance tests can be classified into two groups: walk/run tests or pure walk tests. In the walk/run test, the subject can walk, run, or use a combination of both to complete the test. In the pure walking tests, the subjects are strictly limited to walking (always having one foot on the ground at any given time) the entire test. Another classification for these tests is whether the test is performed over a set distance (e.g., 1 mile) or over a set time period (e.g., 12 minutes). The first test discussed uses a distance of 1.5 miles and requires the subject to complete the distance in the shortest time possible—either by running the whole distance, if possible, or by combining running with periods of walking to offset the fatigue of continuous running in an untrained individual. The second test uses a set 1-mile course and requires the subject to walk the distance.

### 1.5-Mile Run Test Procedures

This test is contraindicated for unconditioned beginners, individuals with symptoms of heart disease, and those with known heart disease or risk factors for heart disease. Your client should be able to jog for 15 minutes continuously to complete this test and obtain a reasonable prediction of their aerobic capacity.

1. Ensure that the area for performing the test measures out to be 1.5 miles in distance. A standard 1/4-mile track would be ideal (6 laps = 1.5 miles).
2. Inform the client of the purposes of the test and the need to pace over the 1.5-mile distance. Effective pacing and the subject's motivation are key variables in the outcome of the test.
3. Have the client start the test; start a stopwatch to coincide with the start. Give your client feedback on time to help them with pacing.
4. Record the total time to complete the test and use the formula below to predict CRF in $mL \cdot kg^{-1} \cdot min^{-1}$.

   For men and women:
   $VO_{2max}$ $(mL \cdot kg^{-1} \cdot min^{-1}) = 3.5 + 483 /$ Time
   Time = time to complete 1.5 miles in nearest hundredth of a minute.

   For example:
   If time to complete 1.5 miles was 11:12 (11 minutes and 12 seconds), then the time used in the formula would be 11.2 (12/60=0.2).
   $VO_{2max}$ $(mL \cdot kg^{-1} \cdot min^{-1}) = 3.5 + 483 / 11.2$
   $= 46.6$ $mL \cdot kg^{-1} \cdot min^{-1}$

## 12-Minute Walk/Run Test Procedures

A popular variation of the 1.5-Mile Run Test is the 12-Minute Walk/Run Test popularized by Dr. Ken Cooper of the Aerobics Institute in Dallas, TX. This test requires the client to cover the maximum distance in 12 minutes by either walking, running, or using a combination of walking and running. The distance covered in 12 minutes needs to be measured and expressed in meters.

The prediction of aerobic capacity from the 12-Minute Walk/Run Test is:

$VO_{2max}$ (mL·kg$^{-1}$·min$^{-1}$) = 3.126 · (meters covered in 12 minutes) − 11.3

## Rockport 1-Mile Walk Test Procedures

This test may be useful for those who are unable to run because of a low fitness level and/or injury. The client should be able to walk briskly (get their exercise HR above 120 bpm) for 1 mile to complete this test.

1. The 1-mile walk test requires that the subject walk 1 mile as fast as they can around a measured course. The client must not break into a run! Walking can be defined as having contact with the ground at all times (running involves an airborne phase). The time to walk this 1 mile is measured and recorded.
2. Immediately at the end of the 1-mile walk, the client counts the recovery HR or pulse for 15 seconds and multiplies by 4 to determine a 1-minute recovery HR (bpm). In another version of the test, HR is measured in the final minute of the 1-mile walk (during the last quarter mile).

The formula for $VO_{2max}$, mL·kg$^{-1}$·min$^{-1}$, is gender specific (i.e., the constant of 6.315 is added to the formula for men only).

$VO_{2max}$ (mL·kg$^{-1}$·min$^{-1}$) = 132.853 − (0.1692 · WT) − (0.3877 · AGE)
   + (6.315, for men) − (3.2649 · TIME) − (0.1565 · HR)

WT = weight in kilograms

AGE = in years

TIME = time for 1 mile in nearest hundredth of a minute (e.g., 15:42
   = 15.7 [42/60=0.7])

HR = recovery HR in bpm

This formula was derived on apparently healthy individuals ranging in age from 30–69 years of age.

For example:

   32-year-old male; 68 kg (150 lbs)
   One mile = 10:35 (10.58); HR = 136
   $VO_{2max}$ (mL·kg$^{-1}$·min$^{-1}$) =
   132.853 − (0.1692 · 68) − (0.3877 · 32) + (6.315) − (3.2649 · 10.58) −
   (0.1565 · 136)
   = 59.4 mL·kg$^{-1}$·min$^{-1}$

## STANDARDS FOR MAXIMUM OXYGEN UPTAKE: $VO_{2max}$ (mL·kg$^{-1}$·min$^{-1}$)

There are several sets of norms for $VO_{2max}$. One set of normative data for maximum oxygen uptake $VO_{2max}$; mL·kg$^{-1}$·min$^{-1}$), found below in Table 6-1, comes from the 6$^{th}$ edition of *ACSM's Guidelines for Exercise Testing and Prescription*.

**TABLE 6.1** PERCENTILE VALUES FOR MAXIMAL AEROBIC POWER (mL•kg⁻¹•min⁻¹)*

| Percentile | Age | | | | |
|---|---|---|---|---|---|
| | **20–29** | **30–39** | **40–49** | **50–59** | **60+** |
| *Men* | | | | | |
| 90 | 51.4 | 50.4 | 48.2 | 45.3 | 42.5 |
| 80 | 48.2 | 46.8 | 44.1 | 41.0 | 38.1 |
| 70 | 46.8 | 44.6 | 41.8 | 38.5 | 35.3 |
| 60 | 44.2 | 42.4 | 39.9 | 36.7 | 33.6 |
| 50 | 42.5 | 41.0 | 38.1 | 35.2 | 31.8 |
| 40 | 41.0 | 38.9 | 36.7 | 33.8 | 30.2 |
| 30 | 39.5 | 37.4 | 35.1 | 32.3 | 28.7 |
| 20 | 37.1 | 35.4 | 33.0 | 30.2 | 26.5 |
| 10 | 34.5 | 32.5 | 30.9 | 28.0 | 23.1 |
| *Women* | | | | | |
| 90 | 44.2 | 41.0 | 39.5 | 35.2 | 35.2 |
| 80 | 41.0 | 38.6 | 36.3 | 32.3 | 31.2 |
| 70 | 38.1 | 36.7 | 33.8 | 30.9 | 29.4 |
| 60 | 36.7 | 34.6 | 32.3 | 29.4 | 27.2 |
| 50 | 35.2 | 33.8 | 30.9 | 28.2 | 25.8 |
| 40 | 33.8 | 32.3 | 29.5 | 26.9 | 24.5 |
| 30 | 32.3 | 30.5 | 28.3 | 25.5 | 23.8 |
| 20 | 30.6 | 28.7 | 26.5 | 24.3 | 22.8 |
| 10 | 28.4 | 26.5 | 25.1 | 22.3 | 20.8 |

*Data provided by Institute for Aerobics Research, Dallas, TX (1994). Study population for the data set was predominately white and college educated. A modified Balke treadmill test was used with $\dot{V}O_{2max}$ estimated from the last grade/speed achieved. The following may be used as descriptors for the percentile rankings: well above average (90), above average (70), average (50), below average (30), and well below average (10).

## SUMMARY

CRF is an important component of health-related physical fitness. CRF is known by many different terms (e.g., maximal aerobic capacity). There has been much research to demonstrate the relationship between CRF and various chronic diseases and disabilities. There are multiple assessments associated with the measurement of CRF that are available to the fitness professional. For example, CRF can be assessed with field tests (Rockport 1-Mile Walk Test), submaximal tests (YMCA Submaximal Cycle Ergometer Test), and maximal tests (Bruce Treadmill Maximal Test). The fitness professional will have to decide which assessment is best for a client and the testing situation. This chapter and the next two chapters discuss some of the various CRF tests to help with this decision.

## LABORATORY EXERCISES

Have all subjects perform all the following three field tests (make sure you allow for adequate recovery between tests—at least 2 hours) to compare the results among the different tests:

- Step Test: McArdle Step Test
- Rockport 1-Mile Walk Test
- 1.5-Mile Run Test

Note: It will be more interesting if you can have these same subjects also perform a laboratory submaximal exercise test (such as the YMCA Submaximal Cycle Ergometer Test) to compare the results to the field tests.

*Suggested Readings*

1. Golding LA, Myers CR, Sinning WE, eds. Y's Way to Physical Fitness, 3rd ed. Champaign, IL: Human Kinetics, 1989.
2. Heyward V. Advanced Fitness Assessment and Exercise Prescription, 3rd edition. Champaign, IL: Human Kinetics, 1998.
3. Howley E, Franks B. Health Fitness Instructor's Handbook, 3rd ed. Champaign, IL: Human Kinetics, 1997.
4. Nieman D. Fitness and Sports Medicine: A Health-Related Approach, 4th ed. Mountain View, CA: Mayfield, 1999.
5. Kline GM, Porcari JP, Hintermeister R, et al. Estimation of $VO_{2max}$ from a 1-mile track walk, gender, age, and body weight. Med Sci Sports Exer 1987;19:253–259.

# 7

# Laboratory Submaximal Exercise Testing:
## *YMCA Cycle Ergometer Test, Åstrand Cycle Ergometer Test, and the Bruce Submaximal Treadmill Test*

Cardiorespiratory fitness (CRF) may be predicted using several testing methodologies that can vary from submaximal to maximal as discussed in Chapter 6. This chapter will discuss the approach of laboratory submaximal exercise testing for predicting maximal aerobic capacity or CRF, as it is a fairly popular approach for CRF testing. Maximal testing is not always a feasible or desirable approach in some settings; therefore, the fitness professional will likely need to be able to perform submaximal exercise tests on a client in a laboratory setting.

A brief review of the advantages and disadvantages of laboratory submaximal exercise testing is worth noting (Box 7-1).

There are several protocols that may be used to conduct a laboratory submaximal exercise test for the prediction of CRF using a variety of testing modalities from the bench step to the cycle to the treadmill. We will discuss the Åstrand protocol and the YMCA protocol used with the cycle ergometer and the Bruce submaximal protocol used with the treadmill (step tests were discussed in the last chapter).

The YMCA (with the help of a group of exercise physiologists) developed a popular protocol with a multistage format that assesses CRF using a cycle ergometer (cycle, not bicycle—the cycle has only one wheel).

---

**BOX 7-1    Advantages and Disadvantages of Laboratory Submaximal Exercise Testing**

*Advantages*
• Relatively inexpensive and require less equipment, personnel, and medical supervision than do maximal exercise tests
• Allows for more mass exercise testing
• Generally shorter test duration time
• If multistage test: can assess multiple HR and BP responses to standardized work outputs

*Disadvantages*
• Maximal measurements (HR, BP $VO_2$) are not taken, but often predicted
• $VO_{2max}$ prediction error can range around 10–20%
• Limited diagnostic utility for certain diseases such as coronary heart disease
• Limited for exercise prescription purposes with no measured $HR_{max}$

Another purpose of the YMCA protocol, or any submaximal test, is the monitoring and evaluation of HR and BP during the defined submaximal work outputs. The submaximal heart rate and blood pressure responses to different work outputs can give information, although limited, concerning the client's cardiovascular system's function and/or efficiency.

Per Olaf Åstrand (a famous exercise physiologist from Sweden), along with his wife, Irma Ryhming, developed a simpler protocol in the 1950s to be used for the prediction of CRF from laboratory submaximal cycle exercise results; this protocol is sometimes known as the Åstrand-Ryhming protocol. This protocol uses a single stage approach for the prediction of CRF. While this protocol is not used as often as the YMCA protocol, it is presented in this manual since it is somewhat simpler to use and may represent a good first protocol to use as the fitness professional learns how to conduct laboratory submaximal exercise tests.

For all practical purposes, the cycle ergometer is the mode of choice for laboratory submaximal testing (as opposed to the treadmill or bench step) because of the exact reproducibility of work output on the cycle ergometer. There are also laboratory submaximal exercise tests, however, that use the treadmill as the test mode. One such protocol uses the traditional Bruce protocol (discussed in Chapter 8, used in maximal exercise testing), but modifies the protocol to be submaximal. This approach is similar to the submaximal cycle protocols discussed earlier in that the goal is to predict CRF.

## DEFINING SUBMAXIMAL TESTING

- Ergometry: is the measurement of work output during a standardized work or exercise test. The cycle ergometer is very useful in exercise testing because it allows for the exact quantification of work output that is a necessary component of ergometry.
- Submaximal Exercise Tests: require that the client who is exercising on a particular mode is doing so at a known work output that is less than their maximal effort. The individual's heart rate for that particular work output is then used to predict CRF. The cycle ergometer provides a more exact quantification of work than other comparable exercise testing modes, like the treadmill. The ability to determine or calculate the exact work output on the cycle ergometer is important to the fitness professional.

## Submaximal Cycle Ergometry Calculations

### Work Output

Work Output $(kp \cdot m \cdot min^{-1})$ = Resistance (kp) $\cdot$ Revolutions per minute (rpm) $\cdot$ Flywheel travel distance [Meters per revolution $(m \cdot rev^{-1})$]

- Work Output $(kp \cdot m \cdot min^{-1})$: total amount of work [Work = Force $\cdot$ Distance]. Work output on the cycle ergometer is often expressed as $kp \cdot m \cdot min^{-1}$. Work output can also be expressed as work rate or workload. This is the basic unit of work on the cycle ergometer; it is difficult to discuss work rates on other modes of exercise (such as the treadmill) in the same way.

     $kp \cdot m \cdot min^{-1}$ = kilopound meter per minute
     $kp \cdot m \cdot min^{-1}$ is nearly synonymous with $k \cdot gm \cdot min^{-1}$.

- Resistance is resistance on flywheel by pendulum weight and friction belt, measured in kilopounds (kp) or kilograms (kg). A kp is the force the swinging pendulum weight applies to the friction belt on the flywheel of the cycle, also called resistance. Resistance can be increased during the test to apply standardized work outputs to the client. Since kp and kg are somewhat interchangeable, the measure of work on the cycle ergometer can also be expressed as k·gm·min$^{-1}$.

- Revolutions per minute (cadence) are simply the number of pedal revolutions per minute (rpm). The YMCA protocol and the Åstrand protocol each call for a constant rpm (very important) of 50 rpm (as do many submaximal cycle protocols). Newer ergometers most likely have an electronic console that can measure cadence or rpm; otherwise, you can set a metronome at 100 bpm (100 bpm for each individual leg = 50 rpm for both legs) to achieve 50 rpm (if the cycle has a tachometer, the appropriate reading would be 18 km·hr$^{-1}$).

- Flywheel travel distance (meters per revolution) is a constant for each type of cycle. The most popular cycle ergometer is the Monark (Vansbro, Sweden). The Monark cycle ergometer has a 6m·rev$^{-1}$ ratio. This means that the flywheel on the Monark cycle will travel 6 meters per complete revolution of the pedal (the flywheel is 1.62 m in circumference and travels 3.7 circuits per pedal revolution). Some models of the Tunturi (Turku, Finland) and Bodyguard (Sandnes, Norway) ergometers each have a 3m·rev$^{-1}$ ratio.

Work outputs, for example:

300 kp·m·min$^{-1}$ = 1 kp · 50 rpm · 6 m·rev$^{-1}$
600 kp·m·min$^{-1}$ = 2 kp · 50 rpm · 6 m·rev$^{-1}$
720 kp·m·min$^{-1}$ = 2 kp · 60 rpm · 6 m·rev$^{-1}$

By using a basic principle of algebra, you may solve for any part of the equation if you know the other parts. For example:

900 kp·m·min$^{-1}$  = X kp · 50 rpm · 6 m·rev$^{-1}$

$$\frac{900 \text{ kp·m·min}^{-1}}{50 \text{ rpm} \cdot 6 \text{ m·rev}^{-1}} = X \text{ kp}$$

3  = kp

### Watts

Finally, work output on the cycle ergometer may also be expressed in Watts, a more scientific unit. Watts can be determined from kp·m·min$^{-1}$ by dividing by 6.1; or dividing by 6 to simplify the conversion. For example, 600 kp·m·min$^{-1}$ is approximately equal to 100 Watts. Note, in the current edition of *ACSM's Metabolic Calculations*, the term Watts is used for work output on the cycle ergometer. Newtons and joules are two other (though less common) ways to express work output.

## CYCLE ERGOMETER

Generally, the Monark cycle ergometer is the most popular brand of "laboratory" cycle because the Monark cycle ergometer allows for accurate and reliable work outputs for the different stages of a submaximal test. There are other ergometer brands that may be used, such as the Tunturi and Bodyguard brands. One potential drawback to using the Monark is the cost of the Monark ergometers.

## Advantages of Cycle Ergometry in Exercise Testing

There are several advantages to using the cycle ergometer for submaximal prediction of CRF rather than other modes of exercise, such as the treadmill. One advantage to the cycle is it is a non-weight bearing mode of exercise, which makes it a good choice for orthopedic injury cases. Also, the cycle ergometer provides accurate workloads that more precisely allow for the prediction of CRF. It is also easier to measure the BP and HR by palpation during exercise because of the limited noise that the cycle ergometer produces and the stabilization of the upper body and arm. The cost of a cycle ergometer is lower than the cost of a treadmill, requires little space, and has no electrical needs.

In summary, the advantages include:

- Non-weight bearing
- Accurate workloads
- Easier to obtain some measurements such as BP and HR palpation
- Cheaper in cost than some other modes

## Disadvantages of Cycle Ergometry in Exercise Testing

There are potential drawbacks to using the cycle ergometer. The cycle is a generally non-familiar work mode, especially in older populations and especially in the United States. More individuals are used to the mode of walking than the mode of cycling. The cycle ergometer demands that the client concentrate to maintain the work output for a stage by maintaining their cadence. Also, a Monark cycle ergometer (or any ergometer that is designed for exercise testing) may not be a very desirable mode for exercise training because it has very few of the "bells and whistles" that clients may desire for routine exercise training. Finally, the treadmill is believed to give a truer physiological max than the cycle ergometer. Your decision to use a cycle ergometer for exercise testing, whether submaximal or maximal, is based on several factors. The fitness professional must carefully weigh the options.

## SUBMAXIMAL PREDICTION OF CARDIORESPIRATORY FITNESS (CRF)
### Assumptions

There are several assumptions that one must make when predicting CRF from submaximal results. With prediction there is error and certain assumptions must be accepted; also if a submaximal treadmill protocol is used to predict CRF, then the assumptions made are similar to the list below, just more tailored for the treadmill than the cycle.

- Between a HR of 110–150 bpm, everyone has a linear (straight line) relationship between $VO_2$ and HR. This is a fairly robust assumption, meaning that it is largely true. In exercise physiology, we know that once the stroke volume has reached a 'plateau' (around 40–50% of max), the HR and $VO_2$ track linearly.
- Maximum heart rate ($HR_{max}$), which must be predicted for submaximal ergometer testing, can be estimated or predicted, since it is a function of age (i.e., $HR_{max} = 220 - age$). Unfortunately, there is a large standard deviation for the age-prediction of $HR_{max}$ and this assumption may provide for the greatest error in submaximal ergometer prediction of CRF.
- Steady state heart rate ($HR_{ss}$)—a steady physiological response—can be achieved in 3 to 4 minutes at a constant, submaximal work output. This is a largely achievable assumption by ensuring that a client reaches a steady state during each and every stage of the protocol chosen. Thus, the achievement of $HR_{ss}$ during the protocol is a very important concept and goal during any submaximal prediction of CRF test.
- The cadence of 50 revolutions per minute (rpm) is comfortable and all are mechanically efficient at this cadence. Most everybody is mechanically efficient at a 50-rpm

cadence, although some may not be comfortable at this cadence. Everyone expends the same amount of energy and has the same absolute oxygen requirements at the same work output on the cycle. This assumption is the basis for *ACSM's Metabolic Calculations*.

- Submaximal work outputs can predict maximal work output and thus maximal aerobic capacity, or $VO_{2max}$. This assumption is a part of the next assumption.
- The HR at two separate work outputs can be plotted as the $HR - VO_2$ relationship and extrapolated to the estimated $HR_{max}$. The YMCA submaximal cycle ergometer protocol and the Bruce submaximal treadmill protocol both are multistage tests that use the concept of at least two stages to predict CRF. The Åstrand protocol is only a single-stage test; this assumption does not directly apply to it.

## Sources of Error in Submaximal Prediction

Along with the assumptions that must be made with submaximal prediction of CRF, there are the sources of error. These sources of error again relate more to the use of the cycle ergometer.

- Prediction (by age; $220 - $ age) of $HR_{max}$.
- Efficiency of the client, or cyclist, on ergometer.
- Calibration of cycle, often taken for granted. It is vital to the accuracy of the test results.
- Accurate measurement of HR during each stage.
- Having a $HR_{ss}$ at each stage.

## SUBMAXIMAL EXERCISE TESTING
## Test Termination Criteria

The conduct of any laboratory submaximal exercise test requires a set of predetermined exercise test endpoints and a satisfactory completion of the test. Given the nature of laboratory submaximal exercise tests, these tests will likely be performed on low- to moderate-risk individuals, based on ACSM guidelines for risk stratification. The general indications for stopping an exercise test in low-risk adults by ACSM should be used (Box 7-2). In addition to this list, you should consider adding a test termination criteria of the client reaching 85% of their age-predicted $HR_{max}$ rate (70% of heart rate reserve). If the client reaches above this 85% of $HR_{max}$, the test is then no longer likely to be submaximal. The *ACSM's Guidelines for Exercise Testing and Prescription* (*ACSM's GETP*) suggests that if the 85% of $HR_{max}$ is exceeded, then the test should be considered maximal with new considerations for a medical examination before and physician supervision of the test as discussed in Chapter 2.

Perform ACSM risk stratification on a client first. Follow the guidelines for the conduct of laboratory submaximal exercise test and physician supervision as discussed in Chapter 2.

## Cycle Calibration

The calibration of the cycle ergometer is the first step and a very important step before performing a laboratory submaximal cycle exercise test. For the Monark Cycle Static Calibration: (Treadmill calibration is not covered in this manual as it varies between treadmill models—see Chapter 8.)

| BOX 7-2 | **General Indications for Stopping an Exercise Test in Low-Risk Adults\*** |
|---------|---------------------------------------------------------------------------|

- Onset of angina or angina-like symptoms.
- Significant drop (20 mm Hg) in systolic blood pressure or a failure of the systolic blood pressure to rise with an increase in exercise intensity.
- Excessive rise in blood pressure: systolic pressure > 260 mm Hg or diastolic pressure > 115 mm Hg.
- Signs of poor perfusion: light-headedness, confusion, ataxia, pallor, cyanosis, nausea, or cold and clammy skin.
- Failure of heart rate to increase with increased exercise intensity.
- Noticeable change in heart rhythm.
- Subject requests to stop.
- Physical or verbal manifestations of severe fatigue.
- Failure of the testing equipment.

\*Assumes that testing is nondiagnostic and is being performed without direct physician involvement or electrocardiographic monitoring.

1. Zero the ergometer by unfastening the resistance belt from the pendulum (note: the ergometer should be on a level surface). Make sure you have adjusted the pendulum resistance lever back to near its starting point.
2. Have your client sit on the cycle, but do not let the feet touch the pedals, which would provide metal stress to the frame.
3. Examine the resistance belt and flywheel for excessive wear and dirt — both the belt and flywheel should be clean. The flywheel can be cleaned with steel wool and cleanser and the belt can also be cleaned with a mild detergent; however, you should not conduct a test if either is wet, so plan ahead. Most resistance belts have a lifespan of several years before they need replacing depending on usage.
4. Check to see that the resistance scale (on the side of the cycle) reads zero; if not, adjust to zero with the thumbscrew.
5. You may add a known weight to the shorter belt (e.g., 1 kg) and check the resistance scale output to ensure that the resistance scale reads that weight (e.g., 1 kg). It is better to attach a heavier calibration weight to magnify any potential error.
6. Finally, re-attach the belt to the mechanism and be sure to pull the belt somewhat tight without too much slack. If you allow for too much slack in the belt when you re-attach the belt, then the resistance mechanism may fail to provide you with the necessary resistance output range (i.e., you will not be able to turn the resistance up to 3 or more kp). Likewise, if you pull the belt too tight, the cycle will not be able to be freewheeled. Check the Monark ergometer handbook to learn more about calibration of the cycle.

## General Procedures for Laboratory Submaximal Exercise Testing

A general summary of the essential procedures for conducting any laboratory submaximal exercise test can be found in *ACSM's GETP* and in Box 7-3.

| BOX 7-3 | **General Procedures for Laboratory Submaximal Exercise Test for Cardiorespiratory Fitness Using a Cycle Ergometer** |
|---|---|

1. The exercise test should begin with a 2- to 3-min warm-up to acquaint the client with the cycle ergometer and prepare him or her for the exercise intensity in the first stage of the test.
2. The specific protocol consists of 3-min stages with appropriate increments in work rate.
3. The client should be properly positioned on the cycle ergometer (i.e., upright posture, 5° bend in the knee at maximal leg extension, hands in proper position on handlebars).
4. Heart rate should be monitored at least 2 times during each stage, near the end of the second and third minutes of each stage. If heart rate > 110 beats·min$^{-1}$, steady state heart rate (i.e., 2 heart rates within 6 beats·min$^{-1}$) should be reached before the work rate is increased.
5. Blood pressure should be monitored in the later portion of each stage and repeated (verified) in the event of a hypotensive or hypertensive response.
6. Perceived exertion should be monitored near the end of each stage using either the 6–20 or the 0–10 scale.
7. Client appearance and symptoms should be monitored regularly.
8. The test should be terminated when the subject reaches 85% of age-predicted maximal heart rate (70% of heart rate reserve), fails to conform to the exercise test protocol, experiences adverse signs or symptoms, requests to stop, or experiences an emergency situation.
9. An appropriate cool-down/recovery period should be initiated consisting of either:
   a. continued pedaling at a work rate equivalent to that of the first stage of the exercise test protocol or lower; or,
   b. a passive cool-down if the subject experiences signs of discomfort or an emergency situation occurs.
10. All physiologic observations (e.g., heart rate, blood pressure, signs and symptoms) should be continued for at least 4 min of recovery unless abnormal responses occur, which would warrant a longer posttest surveillance period.

## YMCA SUBMAXIMAL CYCLE ERGOMETER TEST PROCEDURES

### Multistage Protocol

In summary, the client performs a multistage protocol based on the response to the first stage. The total test may last from 6 to 12 minutes.

1. Explain the test to your client. Be sure you have adequately screened your client via a Health History Questionnaire and/or a PAR-Q and performed ACSM risk stratification. Note: Physician supervision is not necessary with submaximal testing in low- and moderate-risk adults. More information on this can be found in *ACSM's GETP* and in Chapter 2.
2. In addition, you should have already ensured that your client has followed some basic pre-test instructions for this submaximal test: wearing comfortable clothing; having

plenty of fluids beforehand; avoiding alcohol, tobacco, and caffeine within 3 hours of the test; avoiding strenuous exercise on the day of the test; and having adequate sleep the night before the test. These pre-test instructions were discussed in Chapter 2.

3. Explain informed consent. The safety of this test is reported as > 300,000 tests performed without a major complication. Informed consent was discussed in Chapter 2. It is very important that the client understands that he or she is free to stop the test at any time, but he or she is also responsible for informing you of any and all symptoms that might develop.

4. You should also discuss with your client the concept of your general preparedness to handle any emergencies. The details of general preparedness were discussed in Chapter 2 and include the testing environment and emergency plan/procedures. Also an explanation of the rating of perceived exertion (RPE) scale is warranted at this time (Fig. 7-1). An example of some verbal directions you could read to your client before asking them to use the RPE scale to give a general rating is: "Rate your feelings that are caused by exercise using this scale. The feelings should be general, about your whole body. We will ask you to select one number that most accurately corresponds to your perception of your total body feeling. You can use the verbal qualifiers to help you select your RPE number. There is no right or wrong answer. Use any number that you think is appropriate."

5. Take the baseline or resting measures of HR and BP with your client seated. If necessary, these seated measurements can be performed on the cycle ergometer.

6. Adjust seat height. The knee should be flexed at approximately 5 to 10 degrees in the pedal-down position with the toes on the pedals. Another way to check seat height is to have your client place the heels on the pedals; with the heels on the pedals, the leg should be straight in the pedal-down position. Also, you can align the seat height with you client's greater trochanter, or hip, with your client standing next to the cycle. Most important is for your client to be comfortable with the seat height. Have your client turn the pedals to test for the seat height appropriateness. While pedaling, your client should be comfortable and there should be no rocking of the hips (you can check on hip rocking by viewing your client from behind). Also, be sure your client maintains an upright posture (by adjusting the handlebars, if necessary) and does not grip the handlebars too tight.

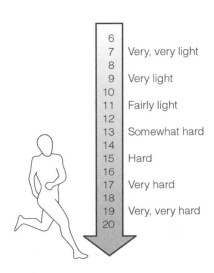

**FIGURE 7-1.** Rating of perceived exertion (RPE) scale.

7. START THE TEST. Have your client freewheel, without any resistance (0 kg), at the pedaling cadence of 50 rpm. A brief period of approximately 2 to 3 minutes should suffice for this freewheeling period. Remember, some subjects may have a difficult time with freewheeling. Maintaining 50 rpm throughout the test is essential. The rpm may vary between ~ 48 and 52 rpm; any more variance than this may invalidate the test.

8. Set the first work output according to YMCA protocol. The first work output, for everyone, is 150 kp·m$^{-1}$·min$^{-1}$ (50 rpm · 0.5 kp). The YMCA protocol is found in Figure 7-2.

## YMCA Submaximal Cycle Ergometer Protocol

9. Start the clock/timer. It may be best to think of timing each stage (e.g., 3 minutes) rather than the entire test time. Therefore, you may wish to reset the time at the end of each stage. In reality, timing of this test is the most difficult part for individuals to learn. Box 7-4 has a suggested timing sequence for each stage of the test.

10. Measure the HR after 2 minutes into the first work rate or stage. Count HR for at least 10 to 15 seconds. Some suggest a 30-second count for more accuracy, however, it may be impractical to spend a full 30 seconds of each minute counting the

|  | | 1st Stage | 150 kgm/min (0.5 kg) |
| --- | --- | --- | --- |

|  | HR < 80 | HR 80–89 | HR 90–100 | HR > 100 |
| --- | --- | --- | --- | --- |
| 2nd Stage | 750 kgm/min (2.5 kg)* | 600 kgm/min (2.0 kg) | 450 kgm/min (1.5 kg) | 300 kgm/min (1.0 kg) |
| 3rd Stage | 900 kgm/min (3.0 kg) | 750 kgm/min (2.5 kg) | 600 kgm/min (2.0 kg) | 450 kgm/min (1.5 kg) |
| 4th Stage | 1050 kgm/min (3.5 kg) | 900 kgm/min (3.0 kg) | 750 kgm/min (2.5 kg) | 600 kgm/min (2.0 kg) |

Directions
1. Set the first work rate at 150 kgm/min (0.5 kg at 50 rpm)
2. If the HR in the third minute of the stage is:
    less than (<) 80, set the second stage at 750 kgm/min (2.5 kg at 50 rpm)
    80–89, set the second stage at 600 kgm/min (2.0 kg at 50 rpm)
    90–100, set the second stage at 450 kgm/min (1.5 kg at 50 rpm)
    greater than (>) 100, set the second stage at 300 kgm/min (1.0 kg at 50 rpm)
3. Set the third and fourth (if required) stages according to

**Figure 7-2.** YMCA cycle ergometry protocol. *Resistance settings shown here are appropriate for an ergometer with a flywheel of 6 m/rev.

| BOX 7-4 | **Suggested Stage Procedures for YMCA Submaximal Cycle Ergometer Test** |
|---|---|

| | |
|---|---|
| 0:00–0:45 | Monitor your client's work output (cadence and resistance) |
| 0:45–1:00 | Pulse count for 15 seconds (for practice) |
| 1:00–1:45 | Monitor your client's work output (cadence and resistance) |
| 1:45–2:00 | Pulse count for 15 seconds (2 min HR) |
| 2:00–2:30 | Stage BP check |
| 2:30–2:45 | Stage RPE check |
| 2:45–3:00 | Pulse count for 15 seconds (3 min HR) |

HR. The use of a HR monitor may be helpful; however, it should only be used as a teaching aid to check your results by palpation. Record the HR on the test form.

11. Measure and record the BP one time during each stage; usually after having completed the 2-minute HR of that stage. *ACSM's GETP* for test termination and BP are applicable.

- BP > 260/115 mmHg
- Significant drop (>20 mmHg) in SBP or a failure to rise with an increase in exercise intensity

12. Ask your client for their RPE for that stage. Choose either the 6–20 scale or the 0–11 scale. These scales were discussed earlier. Be sure to monitor your client for general appearance and any symptoms that may develop.

13. Take another HR after the BP and RPE measurements, around 3 minutes into the stage. Record the HR on the appropriate testing data form.
Compare minute 2 HR to minute 3 HR during each stage:
   A. If there is a difference of within 6 bpm consider that work rate or stage finished. Steady state conditions apply.*
   B. If there is a difference of greater than 6 bpm, continue on for another minute (i.e., minute 4 of that stage) and check HR again. Do not change to the next stage until you have a $HR_{ss}$ (difference within 6 bpm). If you fail to have your client achieve a $HR_{ss}$ for a stage, then you may have to discontinue the test and plan to test again on another day. It has been noted that up to 10% of individuals who are tested with this protocol are unable to obtain $HR_{ss}$ in a stage.
   In summary:
   $HR_{ss}$ (within 6 bpm):          Go to step 15
   No $HR_{ss}$ (> 6 bpm) achieved:     Continue stage until $HR_{ss}$

14. Regularly check the work output of the cycle ergometer using the pendulum resistance scale on the side of the ergometer and the rpm of your client. For the resistance, do not use the scale on the top front panel of the cycle ergometer for measurement. Adjust the work output if necessary. Regularly check your client's rpm and correct if necessary.

---

*The most recent edition (6th) of *ACSM's Guidelines for Exercise Testing and Prescription* suggests that a $HR_{ss}$ may be achieved if the HR between 2 successive minutes is within 6 bpm. (This is different than original YMCA procedures that require a within 5 bpm difference.)

15. After completing the first stage of 150 kp.m$^{-1}$·min$^{-1}$, compare your client's HR$_{ss}$ to the protocol sheet. Adjust resistance appropriately for the second stage based on HR response to 1$^{st}$ stage. This is a multistage test; the client will perform at least two stages.

    • You need to obtain HR$_{ss}$ from a stage (within 6 bpm).
    • The test requires completion of at least 2 separate stages with HR$_{ss}$ at each stage.
    • Consider for the test results the 3$^{rd}$ minute HR as the HR$_{ss}$, if it is a steady state (for plotting or calculations) for that stage.
    • These two stages must have HRs between 110 bpm and 85% of age-predicted heart rate (APMHR) to be used in the plotting and calculation of VO$_{2max}$.

16. Allow your client to cool down after the last stage of the protocol is complete. Have your client continue to pedal at 50 rpm and adjust the resistance down to 0.5 to 1 kp for 3 minutes of cool down or recovery. Take your client's HR and BP at the end of the 3-minute active recovery period. Next, allow him or her to sit quietly in a chair for 2 to 3 minutes to continue the recovery process. Be sure to check the HR and BP before allowing them to leave the lab. Hopefully, the HR and BP will approach the resting measures.

    In summary: Essential Procedures; YMCA
    • HR$_{ss}$ (within 6 bpm) at each stage
    • Accurate HR measurement at each stage
    • Accurate work outputs at each stage (calibration, drift)
    • 2 work outputs that have HRs between 110 bpm and 85% of APMHR
    • Accurate plotting of results

## Prediction of CRF or Maximal Aerobic Capacity (VO$_{2max}$) From YMCA Results

There are two methods available with the YMCA protocol:

• a popular plotting or graphing technique as described below
• a calculation-based formula also described in this manual

### Plotting or Graphing Technique

The HR and work outputs can be plotted to predict/estimate maximal aerobic capacity on the YMCA graph provided in Appendix C.

To plot results and obtain the prediction of VO$_{2max}$, draw a straight line connecting the two HR$_{ss}$ and work outputs points. Extrapolate this line up to the age-predicted (220 − age) HR$_{max}$ and drop a perpendicular line down to VO$_2$/work output axis. The VO$_2$ value is in L·min$^{-1}$. This value for VO$_2$ is then the predicted maximal aerobic capacity or VO$_{2max}$ of your client but it is in the units of absolute VO$_{2max}$ in L·min$^{-1}$.

To convert absolute to relative VO$_2$:

1. Multiply by 1000 to obtain mL·min$^{-1}$
2. Divide by your client's body weight in kg to obtain the maximal aerobic capacity in mL·kg$^{-1}$·min$^{-1}$.

Figure 7-3 describes the process of graphing the HR response for prediction of maximal aerobic capacity. This figure also contains an example how the inaccuracy of age-predicted maximal heart rate might influence the results.

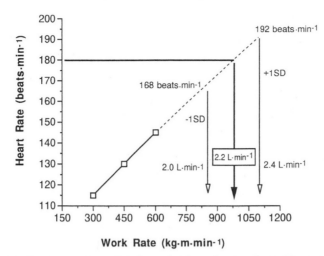

**FIGURE 7-3.** Heart rate responses to 3 submaximal work rates for a 40-year-old, sedentary female weighing 64 kg. $VO_{2max}$ was estimated by extrapolating the heart rate (HR) response to the age-predicted maximal HR of 180 beats·min⁻¹ (based on 220 − age). The work rate that would have been achieved at that HR was determined by dropping a line from that HR value to the x-axis. $VO_{2max,}$ estimated using the formula in Appendix D and expressed in L·min⁻¹, was 2.2 L·min⁻¹. The other 2 lines estimate what the $VO_{2max}$ would have been if the subject's true maximal HR was ± SD from the 180 beats·min⁻¹ value.

## Numerical Calculation of $VO_{2max}$ From the YMCA Test

To predict $VO_{2max}$ from the YMCA Submaximal Cycle Ergometer Test, it is necessary to calculate the slope of the heart rate and $VO_2$ relationship (as is done below) and then calculate the $VO_{2max}$ by using the slope. To predict the maximal aerobic capacity, the following approach would be used:

1. Determine the slope (b) of the HR and $VO_2$:

$$b = \frac{(SM2 - SM1)}{(HR2 - HR1)}$$

   Where:
   SM1 = Submaximal predicted $VO_2$ from stage 1, in mL·kg⁻¹·min⁻¹; see step 2
   SM2 = Submaximal predicted $VO_2$ from stage 2, in mL·kg⁻¹min⁻¹ ; see step 2
   HR1 = $HR_{ss}$, in bpm, from stage 1
   HR2 = $HR_{ss}$, in bpm, from stage 2

2. Determine the SM for each steady-state work output: Use the ACSM Metabolic Calculation Equations for Leg Cycling.
   For cycle workloads between 300 to 1200 kg·m·min⁻¹:
   $VO_2$ (mL·kg⁻¹·min⁻¹) = kg·m·min⁻¹ · 1.8 / BW (kg) + 7

3. Finally, solve the following equation, for $VO_{2max}$, in mL·kg⁻¹·min⁻¹.
   $VO_{2max}$ (mL·kg⁻¹·min⁻¹) = SM2 + b ($HR_{max}$ - HR2)

   where $HR_{max}$ = 220 − age

   For example, a 30-year-old male (75 kg) rode at two stages (450 and 900 kg·m·min⁻¹) and had $HR_{ss}$ of 116 and 130 bpm, respectively. His $VO_{2max}$ would be:

$$b = \frac{(SM2 - SM1)}{(HR2 - HR1)}$$

$$b = \frac{(28.6 - 17.8)}{(130 - 116)} \quad (SM1 = 17.8 \text{ mL·kg}^{-1}\text{·min}^{-1} \text{ and } SM2 = 28.6 \text{ mL·kg}^{-1}\text{·min}^{-1})$$

$$= 0.77$$

$$VO_{2max} (\text{mL·kg}^{-1}\text{·min}^{-1}) = SM2 + b (HR_{max} - HR2)$$
$$= 28.6 + 0.77 ((220 - 30) - 130)$$
$$= 74.8 \text{ mL·kg}^{-1}\text{·min}^{-1}$$

## ÅSTRAND SUBMAXIMAL CYCLE ERGOMETER TEST PROCEDURES

In summary, the client performs a 6-minute submaximal exercise session on the cycle ergometer. Thus, this is typically a single stage test. The HR response to this session will determine the maximal aerobic capacity by plotting the HR response to this one stage on a nomogram.

The calibration of the cycle ergometer is the same as in the YMCA protocol:

1. Explain the test to your client: same as in the YMCA protocol.
2. Explain informed consent: same as in the YMCA protocol.
3. You should also discuss with your client the concept of your general preparedness to handle any emergencies: same as in the YMCA protocol.
4. Take the baseline or resting measures of HR and BP with your client seated: same as in the YMCA protocol.
5. Adjust seat height: same as in the YMCA protocol.
6. START THE TEST. Have your client freewheel, without any resistance (0 kg), at the pedaling cadence of 50 rpm. **Maintaining 50 rpm throughout the test is essential.**
7. Set the first stage's work output according to protocol table (Table 7-1).
8. Start the clock/timer.
9. Measure the HR after each minute starting at minute 2. Count the HR for 10 to 15 seconds. You may wish to use a heart rate monitor, only as a teaching tool. Record the HR on the test form.
10. Measure and record the blood pressure after the 3-minute HR; ACSM Guidelines for test termination and BP are applicable.

---

**TABLE 7-1** Åstrand Cycle Submaximal Cycle Ergometer Test Initial Workloads

This protocol table is designed as a guide. The protocol is designed to elicit a HR of between 125–170 bpm by 6 minutes. You can adjust the work output as necessary during the test (usually after the first 6 minutes) to achieve a HR in or near this range in your subject.

| Individual | Work Output (kp · m⁻¹ · min⁻¹) |
|---|---|
| Men | |
|   Unconditioned | 300–600 |
|   Conditioned | 600–900 |
| Women | |
|   Unconditioned | 300–450 |
|   Conditioned | 450–600 |
| Poorly Conditioned or Older Individuals | 300 |

11. The 5th and 6th minute HR will be used in the test determination of $VO_{2max}$ as long as there is not more than a 6 beat difference between the two HRs.
    The following applies for $HR_{ss}$:

    - If there is a difference of less than or equal to 6 bpm, then consider the test finished.
    - If there is a difference of greater than 6 bpm, then continue on for another minute and check HR again.

12. Regularly check the work output of the cycle ergometer using the pendulum resistance scale on the side of the ergometer and the rpm of subject. For the resistance, do not use the scale on the top front panel for measurement. Adjust the work output if necessary.

13. Regularly check your client's rpm and correct if necessary.

    The Åstrand protocol requires the following for test completion:
    You need to obtain $HR_{ss}$ from the test with the 5th and 6th minute HR (within 6 bpm). For the best (most accurate) prediction of $VO_{2max}$, the HR should be between 125 and 170 bpm.
    If the HR response to the initial work rate is not above 125 bpm after 6 minutes, then the test is continued for another 6-minute interval by increasing the work rate by 300 $kp \cdot m^{-1} \cdot min^{-1}$ (1 kp).
    The HR at the 5th and 6th minutes, if acceptable to the criteria above, is averaged for the nomogram method.

14. Allow your client to cool down after the protocol is complete. Have your client continue to pedal at 50 rpm and adjust the resistance down to 0.5 to 1 kp for 3 minutes of cool down or recovery. Take your client's HR and BP at the end of the 3-minute active recovery period. Next, allow your client to sit quietly in a chair for 2 to 3 minutes to continue the recovery process. Be sure to check your client's HR and BP before allowing your client to leave the lab. Hopefully, the HR and BP will approach the resting measures.

## Prediction of Maximal Aerobic Capacity ($VO_{2max}$) From Åstrand Results

There are two methods available:

- a popular nomogram technique
- a calculation-based formula

### Nomogram Technique

Plot the HR (average for 5th and 6th minute) on the appropriate gender scale along with the corresponding work rate in $kp \cdot m^{-1} \cdot min^{-1}$ (gender specific). Connect the two points with a straight line and read off the $VO_{2max}$ in $L \cdot min^{-1}$ (Fig. 7-4). Use the correction factor table to correct the $VO_{2max}$ by the person's age (nearest 5 years) (Box 7-5).

For example:
    If the estimated $VO_{2max}$, in $L \cdot min^{-1}$, was 3.65 for a 40-year-old male, the age-corrected $VO_{2max}$ would be 3.03 $L \cdot min^{-1}$ [3.65 · 0.83]

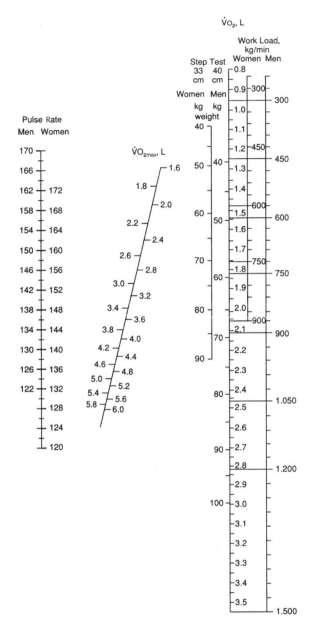

**Figure 7-4.** Modified Åstrand-Ryhming nomogram. Reprinted with permission from Åstrand P-O, Ryhming I. A nomogram for calculation of aerobic capacity (physical fitness) from pulse rate during submaximal work. J Appl Physiol 1954;7:218–221.

## Numerical Calculation of $\dot{V}O_{2max}$ From the Åstrand Protocol

To calculate the $\dot{V}O_{2max}$ in $mL \cdot kg^{-1} \cdot min^{-1}$, from the single stage Åstrand protocol, the following approach can be used:

$$\dot{V}O_{2max} \, (mL \cdot kg^{-1} \cdot min^{-1}) = \frac{SM \cdot (220 - age - 73 - (SEX \cdot 10))}{(HR - 73 - (SEX \cdot 10))}$$

SM = submaximal workload, $VO_2$, in $mL \cdot kg^{-1} \cdot min^{-1}$
SEX = represents 0 for women and 1 for men
HR = steady state HR, in bpm, from submaximal workload

| BOX 7-5 | Age Correction Factor for Åstrand Cycle Ergometer Test Results |
| --- | --- |

| Age | Correction Factor |
| --- | --- |
| 15 | 1.10 |
| 25 | 1.00 |
| 35 | 0.87 |
| 40 | 0.83 |
| 45 | 0.78 |
| 50 | 0.75 |
| 55 | 0.71 |
| 60 | 0.68 |
| 65 | 0.65 |

Determine the SM for the steady state workload: Use the ACSM Metabolic Calculation Equations for Leg Cycling (as described above for the YMCA test)

For cycle workloads between 300 to 1200 $kg \cdot m^{-1} \cdot min^{-1}$:

$VO_2$ $(mL \cdot kg^{-1} \cdot min^{-1})$ = $kg \cdot m \cdot min^{-1} \cdot 1.8 /(kg\ BW) + 7$

For example, a 33-year-old conditioned female (63 kg) rides at 600 $kg.m \cdot min^{-1}$ $(mL \cdot kg^{-1} \cdot min^{-1} = 24.1)$ and has a $HR_{ss}$ = 124 bpm, her

$$VO_{2max}\ (mL \cdot kg^{-1} \cdot min^{-1})\ = \frac{SM \cdot (220 - age - 73 - (SEX \cdot 10))}{(HR - 73 - (SEX \cdot 10))}$$

$$= \frac{24.1 \cdot (220 - 33 - 73 - (0 \cdot 10))}{(124 - 73 - (0 \cdot 10))}$$

$$= \frac{24.1 \cdot (114 - (0))}{(51 - (0))}$$

$$= 53.8\ mL \cdot kg^{-1} \cdot min^{-1}$$

## BRUCE SUBMAXIMAL TREADMILL EXERCISE TEST PROCEDURES

It is possible to conduct laboratory submaximal exercise tests using the treadmill, as opposed to the cycle ergometer. A submaximal treadmill exercise test would also be used to predict CRF. Thus, similar principles and conditions apply to submaximal treadmill exercise test

| TABLE 7-2 | FIRST THREE STAGES OF BRUCE TREADMILL PROTOCOL: SUBMAXIMAL TEST | | |
| --- | --- | --- | --- |
| Stage | Time (min) | Speed (mph) | Grade (%) |
| I | 0–3 | 1.7 | 10 |
| II | 3–6 | 2.5 | 12 |
| III | 6–9 | 3.4 | 14 |

protocols as do submaximal cycle ergometer protocols, such as linear HR-$VO_2$ response and steady state exercise. Note: treadmill calibration will be discussed in the next chapter.

The popular Bruce protocol for treadmill maximal exercise testing can be used for this. The first three stages of the original Bruce protocol are used for this assessment. These first three stages can be found in Table 7-2.

Your client should walk on the treadmill for at least 3 minutes for each stage. Your client's HR would be taken every minute. The concept of $HR_{ss}$ would apply (within 6 bpm). If your client was not at steady state by the 3rd minute (which is very possible), then continue to have your client walk at that same stage for another minute. RPE and BP could also be measured during this protocol, as in the YMCA or Åstrand protocols.

Your client should complete all three stages. The first stage is considered a warm-up stage. The $HR_{ss}$ should be between 115 and 155 bpm (some suggest not allowing the HR to exceed 135 bpm) for the last two stages. To predict the maximal aerobic capacity the following approach would be used:

1. Determine the slope (b) of the HR and $VO_2$:

$$b = \frac{(SM3 - SM2)}{(HR3 - HR2)}$$

Where:

SM2= submaximal $VO_2$ for stage 2
SM3 = submaximal $VO_2$ for stage 3
HR2 = steady state HR for stage 2
HR3 = steady state HR for stage 3
Submaximal $VO_2$ calculations: Treadmill Walking (1.9–3.7 mph)
$VO_2 = [(m \cdot min^{-1}) \cdot 0.1] + [(m \cdot min^{-1}) \cdot 1.8 \cdot grade(decimal)] + 3.5$
$VO_2$ in $mL \cdot kg^{-1} \cdot min^{-1}$
speed conversion: 1 mph = 26.8 $m \cdot min^{-1}$

For example: the submaximal $VO_2$ for the three stages of the Bruce protocol can be found in Table 7-3.

then

$$b = \frac{(34.6 - 25.7)}{(144 - 122)}$$

$b = 0.40$

The $VO_{2max}$ = SM3 + b ($HR_{max}$ − HR3)

where $HR_{max}$ = 220 − age (in this case age = 27; $HR_{max}$ = 193 bpm)

so $VO_{2max}$ = 34.6 + 0.40 (193 − 144)

= 54.2 $mL \cdot kg^{-1} \cdot min^{-1}$

| TABLE 7-3 | EXAMPLE DATA FROM A BRUCE SUBMAXIMAL TREADMILL TEST | |
|---|---|---|
| Stage | $\dot{V}O_2$ (mL·kg⁻¹·min⁻¹) | and, if the HR (bpm) was |
| I (1.7, 10%) | 13.4 | 94 |
| II (2.5, 12%) | 25.7 | 122 |
| III (3.4, 14%) | 34.6 | 144 |

## SUMMARY

The laboratory submaximal assessment of CRF using one of the various protocols available to the fitness professional is one of the more commonly used approaches to CRF assessment. In terms of skill level, it is fairly important to be able to perform these assessments to be certified as an ACSM Health/Fitness Instructor$_{SM}$. The laboratory submaximal assessment can give valuable information about the CRF (both the predicted $VO_{2max}$ and the HR and BP responses to standard amounts of submaximal exercise) of the client. The practice of conducting these assessments will pay great dividends in the ability to conduct a laboratory submaximal CRF assessment, such as the YMCA submaximal cycle ergometer test.

## LABORATORY EXERCISES

1. Have all subjects perform the YMCA Submaximal Cycle Ergometer Test for practice with the test procedures and with the calculation of the results (either or both the graphing solution and the numerical calculation solution). Of course, these could be the same subjects as are used in the Chapter 6 laboratory exercises.
2. Jackie, who weighs 150 pounds, was given a Submaximal Cycle Ergometer test using the YMCA protocol before starting an exercise program. The data from her test is as follows:

   | | |
   |---|---|
   | Age: | 22 yr |
   | Weight: | 150 lbs |
   | 300 kp·m·min$^{-1}$: | HR 132 bpm (steady-state) |
   | 450 kp·m·min$^{-1}$: | HR 146 bpm (steady-state) |

   Plot her data and determine her $VO_{2max}$ in mL·kg$^{-1}$·min$^{-1}$.

   Six months later she was tested again. Her data was:

   | | |
   |---|---|
   | Age: | 23 yr |
   | Weight: | 145 lbs |
   | 300 kp·m·min$^{-1}$: | HR 126 bpm (steady-state) |
   | 450 kp·m·min$^{-1}$: | HR 138 bpm (steady-state) |

   Determine her $VO_{2max}$ in mL·kg$^{-1}$·min$^{-1}$. How do you interpret her results in test #2 as compared to test #1 (consider $VO_{2max}$ and her HR responses)?
3. Sandy was also tested using the YMCA protocol. Her $VO_{2max}$ in L·min$^{-1}$ was estimated to be the same as Jackie's 2nd test. However, her weight is 110 lbs. What is her estimated $VO_{2max}$ in mL·kg$^{-1}$·min$^{-1}$? How does this compare to Jackie's values? How do you explain the difference?
4. Comparing the effect of HR$_{ss}$ differences between multiple tests: determine the CRF, using the YMCA Submaximal Cycle Ergometer Test Results, for the following person:

   Male (165 pounds) and age 45 yrs.

   | Workload | HR (bpm) | | |
   |---|---|---|---|
   | (kpm·min$^{-1}$) | Test 1 | Test 2 | Test 3 |
   | 450 | 124 | 128 | 124 |
   | 600 | 136 | 136 | 140 |

   Determine his $VO_{2max}$ (mL·kg·min$^{-1}$) using age-predicted HR$_{max}$

*Suggested Readings*

1. Golding LA, Myers CR, Sinning WE, eds. Y's Way to Physical Fitness, 3rd ed. Champaign, IL: Human Kinetics, 1989.
2. Heyward V. Advanced Fitness Assessment and Exercise Prescription, 3rd ed. Champaign, IL: Human Kinetics, 1998.
3. Howley E, Franks B. Health Fitness Instructor's Handbook, 3rd ed. Champaign, IL: Human Kinetics, 1997.
4. Nieman D. Fitness and Sports Medicine: A Health-Related Approach, 4th ed. Mountain View, CA: Mayfield , 1999.

# Maximal Exercise Testing

Maximal exercise testing is perhaps the most challenging of all physical fitness assessment tests, not only for the client, but also for the technician(s). Maximal exercise tests are also termed graded exercise tests (GXT) because they are graded by progressively increasing the workload for the client. GXTs have also been referred to as 'stress tests.' The fitness professional, such as an ACSM Health/Fitness Instructor$_{SM}$, may not get involved in conducting GXTs, but undoubtedly should be aware of the GXT process. In planning to conduct a maximal GXT, first consider the situation in which the GXT is to be performed. The following is a partial list of questions that should be considered with reference to a GXT:

1. What is the purpose of a maximal GXT?
2. Who should have a maximal GXT (and current medical examination) before starting a moderate or vigorous exercise program?
3. Should a physician be present to 'supervise' the maximal GXT?
4. What are the personnel needs for conducting the maximal GXT?
5. Which protocol(s) and procedures should be used with a maximal GXT?
6. What are the maximal GXT contraindications and test termination criteria?

Many of these questions are addressed in the most recent edition of *ACSM's Guidelines for Exercise Testing and Prescription* (*ACSM's GETP*). However, it is worth emphasizing again that *ACSM's GETP* represents a collective series of guidelines and opinions. It is up to the clinical judgment of the professional to interpret the guidelines based upon the situation. This chapter will address these six questions.

## 1. WHAT IS THE PURPOSE OF A MAXIMAL GXT?

The maximal GXT has three main purposes:

- Diagnosis of coronary artery disease (CAD) and/or other diseases
- Prognosis of the client, as far as their history with CAD and/or other diseases
- Therapeutic purposes in helping to refine the exercise prescription by providing maximal measurements of functional capacity (cardiorespiratory fitness).

In general, the use of a maximal GXT is more suspect or questioned for the first two purposes of diagnostic or prognostic uses; the application of the maximal GXT to the assessment of functional capacity is more accepted.

## 2. WHO SHOULD HAVE A MAXIMAL GXT (AND CURRENT MEDICAL EXAMINATION) BEFORE STARTING A MODERATE OR VIGOROUS EXERCISE PROGRAM?

*ACSM's GETP* addresses who the candidates are for a GXT by applying the concept of risk stratification. Remember, ACSM risk stratification attempts to answer several questions; one being, "Does a client need a current medical examination and maximal GXT before starting an exercise program?"

Chapter 2 in this manual covered this question in some detail. At this point, it may be important to review the concept that the clients that are low risk and under the age of 45 for men and 55 for women can probably have a submaximal exercise test prior to starting an exercise program according to *ACSM's GTEP*. Clients who are at moderate risk or high risk are recommended to have a maximal GXT with a medical examination before starting a vigorous exercise program.

## 3. SHOULD A PHYSICIAN BE PRESENT TO 'SUPERVISE' THE MAXIMAL GXT?

Another question that the *ACSM's GETP* addresses in the risk stratification area is, "Does a physician need to 'supervise' a submaximal or maximal GXT?"

Chapter 2 in this manual also covered this question. Those clients who are low risk and under the age of 45 for men and under the age of 55 for women can probably have maximal GXT without a physician being present to supervise the test according to *ACSM's GETP*. Clients at moderate risk to high risk are recommended to have a physician be in close proximity to and be readily available to help in any emergency situation that might occur during a maximal GXT.

## 4. WHAT ARE THE PERSONNEL NEEDS FOR CONDUCTING THE MAXIMAL GXT?

The issue of personnel needs to conduct a maximal GXT is not resolved in the literature and is truly based upon the situation. *ACSM's GETP* does not readily address this issue. Other organizations, however, such as the American Heart Association do address personnel needs with a statement about '. . . experienced paramedical personnel . . .' performing maximal GXTs. ACSM does state that

> "... over that past 20 years, cost containment issues and time constraints on physicians have encouraged the use of specially trained health care professionals (e.g., nurses, exercise physiologists, physician assistants, and physical therapists) to administer selected exercise tests, with a physician immediately available for consultation or emergencies that may arise."

This seems to support the notion that a trained and experienced health care professional, such as a fitness professional with the requisite knowledge, skills, and abilities, could administer a maximal GXT. This knowledge, these skills, and these abilities are addressed in Appendix F of *ACSM's GETP*.

When performing a maximal GXT, it would be desirable to have an ACSM certified Exercise Specialist$_{SM}$ present. The relevant sections of *ACSM's GETP* for the performance of a maximal GXT should also be strictly followed, such as the test contraindications, test termination criteria, and emergencies procedures.

## 5. WHICH PROTOCOL(S) AND PROCEDURES SHOULD BE USED WITH A MAXIMAL GXT?

### Protocols

One important preliminary step for performing a maximal GXT is to determine which test protocol to use. An important part of protocol selection is mode selection. For maximal GXTs, the treadmill has traditionally received the most attention because it uses more of the whole body in muscle mass involvement; therefore, the client is able to achieve a greater physiological max than by using, for instance, the cycle ergometer; however, other modes are very possible or desirable. There are many standardized protocols from which to choose. It is also becoming more common to 'individualize' the protocol based on the client, as is discussed further in the chapter.

Generally, the ideal protocol is one in which the client is 'maxed out' or can no longer continue to exercise in around 8–12 minutes (not including warm-up or cool-down). There are two approaches:

| FUNCTIONAL CLASS | CLINICAL STATUS | O₂ COST mL·kg⁻¹·min⁻¹ | METS | BICYCLE ERGOMETER 1 WATT = 6 KPM/MIN (FOR 70 KG BODY WEIGHT, KPM/MIN) | BRUCE 3 MIN STAGES (MPH \ GR) | KATTUS (MPH \ GR) | BALKE-WARE GRADE AT 3.3 MPH 1-MIN STAGES | ELLESTAD 3/2/3 MIN STAGES (MPH \ GR) | USAFSAM (MPH \ GR) | "SLOW" USAFSAM (MPH \ GR) | McHENRY (MPH \ GR) | STANFORD GRADE AT 3 MPH | STANFORD GRADE AT 2 MPH | METS |
|---|---|---|---|---|---|---|---|---|---|---|---|---|---|---|
| NORMAL AND I (HEALTHY, DEPENDENT ON AGE, ACTIVITY) | | 56.0 | 16 | | 5.5 \ 20 ; 5.0 \ 18 | | 26 / 25 | 6 \ 15 | | | | | | 16 |
| | | 52.5 | 15 | | | 4 \ 22 | 24 / 23 | | 3.3 \ 25 | | | | | 15 |
| | | 49.0 | 14 | 1500 | | | 22 / 21 | 5 \ 15 | | | 3.3 \ 21 | | | 14 |
| | | 45.5 | 13 | | 4.2 \ 16 | | 20 / 19 | | 3.3 \ 20 | | | | | 13 |
| | | 42.0 | 12 | 1350 | | 4 \ 18 | 18 / 17 | | | | 3.3 \ 18 | 22.5 | | 12 |
| | | 38.5 | 11 | 1200 | | | 16 / 15 | 5 \ 10 | 3.3 \ 15 | | 3.3 \ 15 | 20.0 | | 11 |
| | | 35.0 | 10 | 1050 | 3.4 \ 14 | 4 \ 14 | 14 / 13 | | | 2 \ 25 | | 17.5 | | 10 |
| | | 31.5 | 9 | 900 | | 4 \ 10 | 12 / 11 | 4 \ 10 | 3.3 \ 10 | 2 \ 20 | 3.3 \ 12 | 15.0 | | 9 |
| | | 28.0 | 8 | 750 | | | 10 / 9 | | | 2 \ 15 | 3.3 \ 9 | 12.5 | | 8 |
| II (SEDENTARY HEALTHY) | | 24.5 | 7 | 600 | 2.5 \ 12 | 3 \ 10 | 8 / 7 | 3 \ 10 | 3.3 \ 5 | 2 \ 10 | 3.3 \ 6 | 10.0 | 17.5 | 7 |
| | | 21.0 | 6 | 450 | | | 6 / 5 | | | 2 \ 5 | | 7.5 | 14 | 6 |
| | | 17.5 | 5 | | 1.7 \ 10 | 2 \ 10 | 4 | 1.7 \ 10 | 3.3 \ 0 | | | 5.0 | 10.5 | 5 |
| III (LIMITED) | | 14.0 | 4 | 300 | | | 3 / 2 | | | 2 \ 0 | 2.0 \ 3 | 2.5 | 7 | 4 |
| | | 10.5 | 3 | | 1.7 \ 5 | | | | | | | 0.0 | 3.5 | 3 |
| | | 7.0 | 2 | 150 | 1.7 \ 0 | | 1 | | 2.0 \ 0 | | | | | 2 |
| IV (SYMPTOMATIC) | | 3.5 | 1 | | | | | | | | | | | 1 |

FIGURE 8-1. Common exercise protocols. Stage I of the conventional Bruce treadmill protocol starts at 1.7 mph, 10% grade. The "modified" Bruce protocol may start at 1.7 mph, 0% grade, or at 1.7 mph, 5% grade, as shown here.

| TABLE 8-1 | THE BRUCE TREADMILL PROTOCOL | | |
|---|---|---|---|
| **Stage** | **Minutes** | **Speed (mph)** | **Grade (%)** |
| I | 1–3 | 1.7 | 10 |
| II | 4–6 | 2.5 | 12 |
| III | 7–9 | 3.4 | 14 |
| IV | 10–12 | 4.2 | 16 |
| V | 13–15 | 5.0 | 18 |
| VI | 16–18 | 5.5 | 20 |

- Use a standardized protocol like the famous Bruce treadmill protocol. The Bruce protocol is popular for graded exercise testing, however, it may not be well suited for testing young healthy individuals or clinical populations like heart patients because it may be too easy or hard for that respective population. It is, however, the most popular GXT protocol in use today.
- Use an individualized protocol designed or customized for the client. From the information attained during the interview with the client, it may be possible to develop an individualized GXT protocol.

Several standardized protocols are presented in Figure 8-1.

## Bruce Treadmill Protocol

Dr. Robert Bruce, a cardiologist, developed the Bruce protocol in the 1960s. The test consists of several 3-minute stages, where the speed and grade are changed each stage, using the treadmill as a mode. Thus, this protocol uses a continuous, progressive approach. There is approximately a 3 MET increase per stage. The protocol starts out at 1.7 mph and 10% grade. As previously mentioned, the protocol tends to be well suited for most middle-aged adults. Generally, heart rate (HR) is measured each minute. Blood pressure (BP) is measured once per stage, usually between the second and third minutes. Rating of perceived exertion (RPE) may also be measured around this time. There is a vast amount of experience and data built up from the use of the Bruce protocol, allowing for easy comparison between subjects, laboratories, and studies. Cardiorespiratory fitness (CRF) can be estimated using several different approaches from a client's performance on the Bruce protocol; this is also discussed in this chapter (Table 8-1).

### One Modification of Bruce Treadmill Protocol

For older or less fit individuals and individuals with CAD, the Bruce protocol has been modified to ease the client's approach into the protocol; however, if you examine the protocol carefully, you will realize that the modification to the protocol is less than complete as it only modifies the first stage of the protocol (Table 8-2).

| TABLE 8-2 | MODIFICATION OF THE BRUCE TREADMILL PROTOCOL | | |
|---|---|---|---|
| **Stage** | **Minutes** | **Speed (mph)** | **Grade (%)** |
| 0 | 1–3 | 1.7 | 0% |
| .5 | 4–6 | 1.7 | 5% |

. . . then proceed into regular Bruce Protocol

## Balke-Ware Treadmill Protocol

Another 'popular' treadmill GXT protocol is the Balke-Ware protocol developed by Dr. Bruno Balke and colleagues. The Balke-Ware protocol has the distinction of being 'modified' by many and in numerous ways. The original Balke-Ware protocol is as follows (Table 8-3):

## Ramp Protocols

A fairly new procedure with treadmill GXTs is to use a ramp protocol instead of the traditional incremental step protocols (Bruce protocol changes speed and grade every 3 minutes in stages). Ramp protocols attempt to more gradually increase the workload by usually shortening the stage time and decreasing the speed and grade increments. Following is an example of a ramp protocol that mimics the Bruce protocol. In this protocol, referred to as the BSU/Bruce ramp protocol, speed and grade change every 20 seconds. Modern equipment (treadmill controllers and electrocardiograph [ECG] machines) is typically needed to conduct ramp protocols (Table 8-4).

## Individualized Protocols

Using an individualized protocol, the general idea is to arrive at a comfortable walking or jogging speed on the treadmill for the client. This then will be the speed used throughout the entire duration of the test. One way to do this:

1. As an orientation to the treadmill, start the treadmill at a walking speed of around 2.0 mph.
2. When your client appears to be comfortable, increase the speed to approach their normal workout speed, if they use the treadmill to exercise. Allow time for your client to adjust to each new treadmill speed. Closely observe your client to ensure that the speed is appropriate. People will often say they walk/jog faster than they really do. If your client reports to exercise outside by walking or running, then convert the exercise routine into a speed (i.e., they walk about 2.5 miles in 50 minutes; that equals 3 mph), then set the speed of the treadmill slower than this speed. Once again, the key is your client's comfort and appearance.
3. For a walking test, use a modified Balke protocol. Stage 1 will start at 0% grade and each stage will increase 2.5% every 2 minutes. How to determine the starting speed and grade for the walking protocol depends on your client's HR. The test should start with a HR of around 100 bpm (Table 8.5).
4. For a running test, minutes 1–4 will be at 0% grade. Minutes 5–6 will be increased to 4% grade, continuing at the same running/walking speed. Minutes 7–8 will be at 6% grade, minutes 9–10 at 8% grade, minutes 11–12 at 10% grade, and so on (Table 8-5)

| TABLE 8-3 | THE BALKE-WARE TREADMILL PROTOCOL | |
|---|---|---|
| Balke-Ware summary: 1-minute stages at a constant speed of 3.3 mph and a 1% grade increase every minute. | | |
| **Minute** | **Speed (mph)** | **Grade (%)** |
| 1 | 3.3 | 1 |
| 2 | 3.3 | 2 |
| 3 | 3.3 | 3 |
| 4 | 3.3 | 4 |
| 5 | 3.3 | 5 |

. . . follow the pattern of a 1% grade increase each minute.

| TABLE 8-4 | THE BALL STATE UNIVERSITY (BSU)/BRUCE TREADMILL RAMP PROTOCOL | | | | | | |
|-----------|------|-------|-------|-------|------|-------|-------|
| **Stage** | **Time** | **Speed** | **Grade** | **Stage** | **Time** | **Speed** | **Grade** |
| 1 | 0:00 | 1.7 | 0.0 | 33 | 10:40 | 4.0 | 15.2 |
| 2 | 0:20 | 1.7 | 1.3 | 34 | 11:00 | 4.1 | 15.4 |
| 3 | 0:40 | 1.7 | 2.5 | 35 | 11:20 | 4.2 | 15.6 |
| 4 | 1:00 | 1.7 | 3.7 | 36 | 11:40 | 4.2 | 16.0 |
| 5 | 1:20 | 1.7 | 5.0 | 37 | 12:00 | 4.3 | 16.2 |
| 6 | 1:40 | 1.7 | 6.2 | 38 | 12:20 | 4.4 | 16.4 |
| 7 | 2:00 | 1.7 | 7.5 | 39 | 12:40 | 4.5 | 16:6 |
| 8 | 2:20 | 1.7 | 8.7 | 40 | 13:00 | 4:6 | 16.8 |
| 9 | 2:40 | 1.7 | 10.0 | 41 | 13:20 | 4.7 | 17.0 |
| 10 | 3:00 | 1.8 | 10.2 | 42 | 13:40 | 4.8 | 17.2 |
| 11 | 3:20 | 1.9 | 10.2 | 43 | 14:00 | 4.9 | 17.4 |
| 12 | 3:40 | 2.0 | 10.5 | 44 | 14:20 | 5.0 | 17.6 |
| 13 | 4:00 | 2.1 | 10.7 | 45 | 14:40 | 5.0 | 18.0 |
| 14 | 4:20 | 2.2 | 10.9 | 46 | 15:00 | 5.1 | 18.0 |
| 15 | 4:40 | 2.3 | 11.2 | 47 | 15:20 | 5.1 | 18.5 |
| 16 | 5:00 | 2.4 | 11.2 | 48 | 15:40 | 5.2 | 18.5 |
| 17 | 5:20 | 2.5 | 11.6 | 49 | 16:00 | 5.2 | 19.0 |
| 18 | 5:40 | 2.5 | 12.0 | 50 | 16:20 | 5.3 | 19.0 |
| 19 | 6:00 | 2.6 | 12.2 | 51 | 16:40 | 5.3 | 19.5 |
| 20 | 6:20 | 2.7 | 12.4 | 52 | 17:00 | 5.4 | 19.5 |
| 21 | 6:40 | 2.8 | 12.7 | 53 | 17:20 | 5.4 | 20.0 |
| 22 | 7:00 | 2.9 | 12.9 | 54 | 17:40 | 5.5 | 20.0 |
| 23 | 7:20 | 3.0 | 13.1 | 55 | 18:00 | 5.6 | 20.0 |
| 24 | 7:40 | 3.1 | 13.4 | 56 | 18:20 | 5.6 | 20.5 |
| 25 | 8:00 | 3.2 | 13.6 | 57 | 18:40 | 5.7 | 20.5 |
| 26 | 8:20 | 3.3 | 13.8 | 58 | 19:00 | 5.7 | 21.0 |
| 27 | 8:40 | 3.4 | 14.0 | 59 | 19:20 | 5.8 | 21.0 |
| 28 | 9:00 | 3.5 | 14.2 | 60 | 19:40 | 5.8 | 21.5 |
| 29 | 9:20 | 3.6 | 14.4 | 61 | 20:00 | 5.9 | 21.5 |
| 30 | 9:40 | 3.7 | 14.6 | 62 | 20:20 | 5.9 | 22.0 |
| 31 | 10:00 | 3.8 | 14.8 | 63 | 20:40 | 6.0 | 22.0 |
| 32 | 10:20 | 3.9 | 15.0 | | | | |

From Kaminsky LA, Whaley MH. Evaluation of a new standardized ramp protocol: the BSU/Bruce Ramp Protocol. J Cardiopulm Rehabil 1998;18:438–444.

For this protocol CRF can be estimated by the following equation:

$$\dot{V}O_{2max}\ (mL \cdot kg^{-1} \cdot min^{-1}) = 3.9\ (test\ time) - 7.0$$

| TABLE 8-5 | EXAMPLE OF AN INDIVIDUALIZED TREADMILL WALKING OR RUNNING PROTOCOL | | | | | |
|-----------|------|-------|-----------|------|-------|-----------|
| | **Walking** | | | **Running** | | |
| **Min** | **Speed** | **Grade (%)** | | **Min** | **Speed** | **Grade (%)** |
| 0– 2 | walking: constant | 0 | | 0–4 | running: constant | 0 |
| 3–4 | | 2.5 | | 5–6 | | 4 |
| 5–6 | | 5 | | 7–8 | | 6 |
| 7–8 | | 7.5 | | 9–10 | | 8 |
| 9–10 | | 10 | | 11–12 | | 10 |
| etc. | | | | etc. | | |

This discussion serves only as a guideline for these protocols. Modifications will be needed based on the client's appearance, performance, BP, and HR responses throughout the test.

## Generalized Procedures

There are several generalized procedures that should be conducted during a graded exercise test. A list of the generalized procedures may be found in Box 8-1.

There are several roles or tasks that need to be performed (and, therefore, several technicians needed) during the administration of a maximal GXT. These roles and tasks are listed in this manual as an example of how an exercise test laboratory might coordinate the tasks that need to be performed. These job descriptions may not be consistent from lab to lab. The following roles are possibly needed:

- Test operator
- ECG technician
- BP technician

### Role of the Test Operator

As the test operator, you are 'in charge' of the GXT.

1. Check emergency equipment in the laboratory before the testing session starts, e.g., defibrillator, emergency drug box, oxygen, suction, airway. (*ACSM's GETP* Appendix B has detailed information on emergency preparation and procedures.)

---

**BOX 8-1** | **Sequence of Measures for HR, BP, RPE, and Electrocardiogram (ECG) During Exercise Testing**

*Pretest*
1. 12-lead ECG in supine and exercise postures
2. Blood pressure measurements in the supine position and exercise posture

*Exercise**
1. 12-lead ECG recorded during last 15 seconds of every stage and at peak exercise (3-lead ECG observed/recorded every minute on monitor)
2. Blood pressure measurements should be obtained during the last minute of each stage[†]
3. Rating scales: RPE at the end of each stage, other scales if applicable

*Posttest*
1. 12-lead ECG immediately after exercise, then every 1 to 2 minutes for at least 5 minutes to allow any exercise-induced changes to return to baseline
2. Blood pressure measurements should be obtained immediately after exercise, then every 1 to 2 minutes until stabilized near baseline level
3. Symptomatic ratings should be obtained using appropriate scales as long as symptoms persist after exercise

---

*In addition, these referenced variables should be assessed and recorded whenever adverse symptoms or abnormal ECG changes occur. Note: An unchanged or decreasing systolic blood pressure with increasing workloads should be retaken (i.e., verified immediately).

[†]Note: An unchanged or decreasing systolic blood pressure with increasing workloads should be retaken (i.e., verified immediately).

2. Review emergency procedures.
3. Check treadmill operation. If the treadmill has been moved or unplugged or a power outage has occurred, then it should be re-calibrated. Treadmill calibration procedures vary from model to model, so check the equipment manual for that particular treadmill for more information. Check the position of treadmill and correct, if necessary.
4. Review client's file. Choose a protocol that best suits your client.
5. Meet client: explain the purpose of the test: "to measure how they respond to exercise so an individualized exercise prescription can be developed."
6. Review the client's medical history/health habit questionnaire (see the Health/History Questionnaire in Appendix C)
7. Explain GXT procedure to client:

    • Walking/running on treadmill: a comfortable walking/running speed will be achieved, than the speed and/or grade will be increased with every stage. Client will be asked if they can go up in slope/grade before each increase.
    • Monitoring HR, BP, ECG, RPE.
    • Client should perform as much work as they possibly can. Make sure they understand that the GXT is maximal.
    • Some risk involved, but emphasize that the risk will be minimized.
    • Client is free to stop the test, at any time, if they wish.
    • Explain the RPE scale (see Chapter 7)

8. Perform informed consent.
9. Ask if they have any questions; tell them they are free to ask questions at any time.
10. After client has been prepped and resting data has been collected, turn on the treadmill and demonstrate how to walk on the treadmill. The BP technician, if you have one, can help to orient the client with the treadmill.
11. Have client get on the treadmill. After they feel comfortable on the treadmill, advance the treadmill speed to the first stage of the test. If the protocol is individualized for your client, the speed should be fast but comfortable enough to complete the test. This also serves as a warm-up for your client. The HR should be around 100 bpm for the initial stage.
12. Watch your client closely. Talk with your client about the work rate. Ask only YES/NO questions, try not to confuse your client with many open-ended questions.
13. Instruct the BP technician and ECG technician, if you have them, when readings should be taken, and that they must voice them to you (loudly and clearly).
14. Record HR, BP, and RPE on the test data form.
15. Continue to increase your client through the protocol by increasing work rates at the set interval according to the protocol. Make sure that your client gives consent to each work rate increase.
16. Talk with your client frequently and offer encouragement to motivate the client to continue.
17. When the test ends (client requests or test termination criteria), decrease the percent grade and speed of treadmill quickly. Ask your client about the reason for stopping the test. Keep your client walking, if possible, and make sure treadmill speed is adequate (2.0–2.5 mph) to maintain blood flow back to heart.
18. Record recovery measures (i.e., HR and BP) each minute.
19. Perform appropriate recovery (e.g., 5 minutes of walking, 2–3 minutes of sitting).
20. Explain post-test procedures:

    • Lukewarm shower (not hot nor cold)
    • Drink water

- No heavy meal for 1 hour
- No heavy exercise or physical activity for the remainder of the day

Help your client get unhooked from the ECG wires and electrodes. Help him or her off the treadmill and take another BP reading (about 2 minutes later) before releasing the client from the lab.

## Role of the ECG Technician

With the advent of fully automated, computerized ECG-treadmill testing systems, there may be less of a need for a separate ECG technician.

1. Turn on the ECG machine.
2. Check the calibration of the ECG machine and paper supply.
3. Check electrodes, lead wires, and prep equipment.
4. When the test operator has finished explaining procedures, prep the client for the ECG in the supine position.
5. Record resting 12-lead ECG in the supine position.
6. Record standing resting ECG.
7. Help client over to treadmill.
8. Check shoelaces and pant legs (if wearing pants) for safety before they get on the treadmill.
9. When the test starts, record HR/ECG every minute. Watch the monitor closely throughout test.
10. When the test ends (know ECG termination points—you may have to advise test operator of termination of test because of ECG changes), record HRmax.
11. Watch the ECG monitor closely and record HR/ECG every minute during recovery. When your client has fully recovered, remove the cable and electrodes.

## Role of the BP Technician

1. Wrap BP cuff around client's arm (check for appropriate cuff—see Chapter 3). It may be helpful to tape the cuff to the client's arm.
2. Take resting supine and standing BP.
3. Explain and demonstrate how to get on and walk on the treadmill.
   - Straddle treadmill belt with feet
   - Lead with heel of foot in front of body
   - Take long, normal strides
   - Look forward and keep head up
   - Let go of handrails when comfortable
4. Help client onto treadmill.
5. During the test, stand close by and talk to client. You will serve as a spotter in case the client falls during the test. Note signs and symptoms the client may experience.
6. Take BP near the end of each stage, and voice the measurement so the test operator can record it. Respond to the test operator's request for additional BP measurements. BP may not be able to be taken when the client starts to run on treadmill.
7. When test ends, take a BP as soon as possible. This is termed the immediate post exercise BP.
8. Help client, if unsteady, into an active (walking) recovery.
9. Take BP each minute of walking recovery.

10. When treadmill has stopped, help the client to sit down. Take BP immediately.
11. If the client has recovered and the test operator has terminated the test, remove the BP cuff.

## 6. WHAT ARE THE MAXIMAL GXT CONTRAINDICATIONS AND TEST TERMINATION CRITERIA?

When performing maximal GXTs, it is important to have clear guidelines for the medical conditions that may exclude a client from performing a maximal GXT for safety reasons. These are known as contraindications. Also, the specific responses that a client may exhibit during the maximal GXT that would cause the test to be terminated early (before the volitional fatigue) are known as test termination criteria. *ACSM's GETP* addresses the contraindications (Box 8-2) and the test termination criteria (Box 8-3). It is interesting that both of these guidelines are separated into absolute and relative areas. Absolute, for both contraindications and test termination criteria, means that a maximal GXT should not be conducted (contraindicated) or should be immediately stopped (test termination) if any of these conditions or responses are exhibited by the client. Relative, on the other hand, allows for clinical judgment in that a maximal GXT may be performed or continued if the benefit of performing the test outweighs the safety or risk exhibited by the client. Relative contraindications (Box 8-2) and test termination criteria (Box 8-3) may be beyond the scope of the fitness professional, or any paramedical professional, to decide on the relative merits for contraindication or test termination.

## 7. PREDICTION OF MAXIMAL AEROBIC CAPACITY ($\dot{V}O_{2MAX}$) FROM BRUCE PROTOCOL PERFORMANCE

A client's CRF can be predicted from their performance on the standardized, popular Bruce protocol for treadmill exercise. Given that the client puts forth a maximal effort (terminated the test at volitional fatigue) during the Bruce GXT then the prediction is possible by using the information of how long they lasted (time) on the protocol; however, it is vital to remember that the client must have given a maximal effort; one in which your client stops the test because of volitional fatigue. In clinical settings, a physician may terminate an exercise test on a client before volitional fatigue because of many factors including responses on the ECG that may indicate ischemia. If the test is terminated before maximal effort, or volitional fatigue, is achieved, then the prediction of CRF is not accurate.

There are three common approaches to predicting CRF from Bruce protocol results:

1. Use of a simple multiplication of the total test time to determine the $\dot{V}O_{2max}$
2. Use of a prediction equation using total test time cubed to determine the $\dot{V}O_{2max}$
3. Use of the MET cost estimates for each minute of the Bruce protocol.

### $\dot{V}O_{2max}$ From Total Test Time (TT)

Select the most appropriate regression formula (men, women, or young men). The $\dot{V}O_{2max}$ in $mL \cdot kg^{-1} \cdot min^{-1} =$

Men: $2.94 \cdot$ Time (min) $+ 7.65$
Women: $2.94 \cdot$ Time (min) $+ 3.74$
Young men: $3.62 \cdot$ Time (min) $+ 3.91$

---

**BOX 8-2** | **Contraindications to Exercise Testing***

*Absolute*
- A recent significant change in the resting ECG suggesting significant ischemia, recent myocardial infarction (within 2 days), or other acute cardiac event
- Unstable angina
- Uncontrolled cardiac arrhythmias causing symptoms or hemodynamic compromise
- Severe symptomatic aortic stenosis
- Uncontrolled symptomatic heart failure
- Acute pulmonary embolus or pulmonary infarction
- Acute myocarditis or pericarditis
- Suspected or known dissecting aneurysm
- Acute infections

*Relative[†]*
- Left main coronary stenosis
- Moderate stenotic valvular heart disease
- Electrolyte abnormalities (e.g., hypokalemia, hypomagnesemia)
- Severe arterial hypertension (i.e., systolic BP of >200 mmHg and/or a diastolic BP of >110 mmHg) at rest
- Tachyarrhythmias or bradyarrhythmias
- Hypertrophic cardiomyopathy and other forms of outflow tract obstruction
- Neuromuscular, musculoskeletal, or rheumatoid disorders that are exacerbated by exercise
- High-degree atrioventricular block
- Ventricular aneurysm
- Uncontrolled metabolic disease (e.g., diabetes, thyrotoxicosis, or myxedema)
- Chronic infectious disease (e.g., mononucleosis, hepatitis, AIDS)

*Modified from Gibbons RA, Balady GJ, Beasely JW, et al. ACC/AHA guidelines for exercise testing. J Am Coll Cardiol 1997;30:260–315.

[†]Relative contraindications can be superseded if benefits outweigh risks of exercise. In some instances, these individuals can be exercised with caution and/or using low-level end points, especially if they are asymptomatic at rest.

---

For example, if a woman lasts 7:52 (52/60 = .86) on the Bruce protocol, then her $\dot{V}O_{2max}$ is:

$$\dot{V}O_{2max}\,(mL \cdot kg^{-1} \cdot min^{-1}) = 2.94 \cdot (7.86) + 3.74$$
$$\dot{V}O_{2max} = 26.8\ mL \cdot kg^{-1} \cdot min^{-1}$$

## Prediction Equation Using Total Test Time Cubed (TT³)

$\dot{V}O_{2max}\,(mL \cdot kg^{-1} \cdot min^{-1}) = 14.8 - 1.379\,(\text{test time}) + 0.451\,(\text{test time}^2) - 0.012\,(\text{test time}^3)$

For example, if the client lasts 8:22, then:

Time $= 8.37$ (22/60)

$T^2 = 70.06$

$T^3 = 586.38$

| BOX 8-3 | Indications for Terminating Exercise Testing* |
|---------|-----------------------------------------------|

*Absolute*
- Drop in systolic blood pressure of 210 mmHg from baseline blood pressure despite an increase in workload, when accompanied by other evidence of ischemia
- Moderate to severe angina
- Increasing nervous system symptoms (e.g., ataxia, dizziness, or near syncope)
- Signs of poor perfusion (cyanosis or pallor)
- Technical difficulties monitoring the ECG or systolic blood pressure
- Subject's desire to stop
- Sustained ventricular tachycardia
- ST elevation ($\geq 1.0$ mm) in leads without diagnostic Q-waves (other than $V_1$ or aVR)

*Relative*
- Drop in systolic blood pressure of $\geq 10$ mmHg from baseline blood pressure despite an increase in workload, in the absence of other evidence of ischemia
- ST or QRS changes such as excessive ST depression (>2 mm horizontal or downsloping ST-segment depression) or marked axis shift
- Arrhythmias other than sustained ventricular tachycardia, including multifocal PVCs, triplets of PVCs, supraventricular tachycardia, heart block, or bradyarrhythmias
- Fatigue, shortness of breath, wheezing, leg cramps, or claudication
- Development of bundle-branch block or intraventricular conduction delay that cannot be distinguished from ventricular tachycardia
- Increasing chest pain
- Hypertensive response[†]

*Reprinted with permission from Gibbons RA, Balady GJ, Beasely JW, et al. ACC/AHA guidelines for exercise testing. J Am Coll Cardiol 1997;30:260–315.

[†]Systolic blood pressure of more than 250 mmHg and/or a diastolic blood pressure of more than 115 mmHg.

$$VO_{2max} = 14.8 - (1.379 \cdot 8.37) + (0.451 \cdot 70.06) - (0.012 \cdot 586.38)$$
$$VO_{2max} = 27.49 \text{ mL} \cdot \text{kg}^{-1} \cdot \text{min}^{-1}$$

## MET Cost Estimates of Each Minute

MET cost of each minute of the Bruce protocol is listed in Table 8-6. For example, if a subject lasts 7 minutes (Stage 3, first minute) the MET cost = 8.3 ($8.3 \cdot 3.5 = 29.05$ mL $\cdot$ kg$^{-1}$ $\cdot$ min$^{-1}$)

## SUMMARY

The GXT for CRF assessment is a vigorous assessment for both the client and the technician compared to something like the Handgrip Assessment for muscular strength. While the GXT is perhaps the most accurate of all the CRF assessments, it also requires the most in terms of equipment, facilities, and technicians. For instance, the choice of using a GXT

**TABLE 8-6** METABOLIC EQUIVALENTS PER MINUTE OF THE BRUCE TREADMILL PROTOCOL

| MIN | METs | MIN | METs | MIN | METs |
|-----|------|-----|------|-----|------|
| 1 | 3.1 | 6 | 7.4 | 11 | 11.6 |
| 2 | 4.0 | 7 | 8.3 | 12 | 12.5 |
| 3 | 4.9 | 8 | 9.1 | 13 | 13.3 |
| 4 | 5.7 | 9 | 10 | 14 | 14.1 |
| 5 | 6.6 | 10 | 10.7 | 15 | 15 |

on the client may require the assistance of a physician should the ACSM Risk Stratification point towards this need. Thus, while the GXT represents the most accurate assessment for CRF, there are several considerations for using it that may not make it the best choice for the client.

## LABORATORY EXERCISES

1. Perform, or participate in performing, five Maximal Treadmill Exercise Tests, using the Bruce Treadmill protocol. Determine the $VO_{2max}$ (mL · kg$^{-1}$ · min$^{-1}$) using the three different methods discussed in this chapter:
   - Using a simple multiplication of the total test time to determine the $VO_{2max}$
   - Using a prediction equation with a total test time cubed to determine the $VO_{2max}$
   - Use of the MET cost estimates for each minute of the Bruce Treadmill protocol.

2. Have three subjects perform the Bruce Treadmill Protocol and the BSU/Bruce Treadmill Protocol (ramp protocol) to compare the procedures and results.

*Suggested Readings*

1. Froelicher V. Exercise and the Heart; Clinical Concepts, 2nd ed. Chicago, IL: Year Book Medical Publishers, 1988.
2. Froelicher V, Marcondes G. Manual of Exercise Testing. Chicago, IL: Year Book Medical Publishers, 1989.
3. Pollock M, Wilmore J. Exercise in Health and Disease: Evaluation and Prescription for Prevention and Rehabilitation, 2nd ed. Philadelphia, PA: WB Saunders, 1990.
4. Wassermann K, Hansen J, Sue D, et al. Principles of Exercise Testing and Interpretation, 2nd ed. Philadelphia, PA: Lea & Febiger, 1994.

# 9

# Interpretation of Assessment Results:
## *Case Studies*

## INTRODUCTION

The assessment of all five components of health-related physical fitness would not be complete without an interpretation of those results. The assessment of an individual's health-related physical fitness can provide valuable information to help develop a safe, effective, and individualized exercise program. The development of an exercise program requires careful consideration to the Medical/Health History and Pre-Activity Screening (including ACSM Risk Stratification), and the individual responses to the selected tests of health-related physical fitness. In this chapter, we will interpret the health-related physical fitness test results for one client, Jane Slimmer. In addition, another set of test results (John Quick) are provided for you to interpret.

As you interpret the various health-related physical fitness test results, remember to consult the specific chapter in this manual that deals with that health-related physical fitness component. In addition, the following summary is provided for you:

- The first step in any assessment of health-related physical fitness is to perform a Pre-Activity Screening including a medical/health history, physical examination, and ACSM risk stratification (this is covered in Chapter 2).
- There are various techniques available to assess body composition including height/weight charts, body mass index, waist-to-hip ratio, and percent body fat (see Chapter 4 for more specific information).
- The assessment of flexibility, muscular strength, and muscular endurance is often grouped together and can occur using several different tests (Chapter 5 contains several tests for each component).
- Cardiorespiratory fitness can be assessed using several techniques that can be classified as either laboratory or field tests for the estimation and/or measurement of $\dot{V}O_{2max}$ (Chapter 6 describes the overall approach to CRF testing).
- There are several submaximal cycle and treadmill protocols that can be used to estimate cardiorespiratory fitness, including the popular YMCA Submaximal cycle test used by many health/fitness professionals (see Chapter 7 for full descriptions).
- Maximal exercise testing using the treadmill and the popular Bruce treadmill graded exercise test may also be used for cardiorespiratory fitness assessment (Chapter 8 discusses this aspect of assessment).

## CASE 1: JANE SLIMMER

Jane Slimmer is a 45-year-old Caucasian woman. Her health-related physical fitness assessment data are provided here; we will analyze the results. This analysis of her health-related physical fitness will necessarily involve many of the other chapters of this manual using several of the tables and figures provided.

### Medical History (Health History Questionnaire)

Ms. Slimmer has no past medical history to report, nor is she currently experiencing any signs and symptoms suggestive of any disease. She reports no family history of major risk factors for cardiovascular disease (e.g., high BP or diabetes). Her 78-year-old mother has osteoporosis. Ms. Slimmer is on estrogen replacement therapy (ERT) following a radical hysterectomy in 2000. She reports no other significant health/medical history on the Health History Questionnaire form. Her interview after she had turned in the Health History Questionnaire was unremarkable.

# Health Behavior Habits (Health History Questionnaire)

Ms. Slimmer denies any experience with sports or recreation. She has been a non-smoker for her whole life. Her occupation of clerk/typist involves almost exclusively sedentary activities on the job. She admits to compulsive feelings towards food. Recently, she has become more interested in weight loss and hopes to regain some of her youthful energy.

On the several health-related physical fitness test data forms, you will find some of her resting and health-related physical fitness assessments results that pertain to classifying

---

### HEALTH HISTORY QUESTIONNAIRE

NAME _Jane_ ___ _Slimmer_   AGE _45_   DATE _10_|_01_|_02_   DATE OF BIRTH _01_|_10_|_57_
First    M.I.    Last                          day / month / yr                day / month / yr

ADDRESS _123_  _Oak Street_   _Activeville_    _PA_   _12345_
          Street              City            State   Zip

TELEPHONE (home) _123-4567_ _____ (Business) _765-4321_ _____

OCCUPATION _Clerk / typist_   PLACE OF EMPLOYMENT _USA Products_ _____

MARITAL STATUS: (circle one)    SINGLE   (MARRIED)   DIVORCED   WIDOWED    SPOUSE: _Bob_

EDUCATION: (check highest level) ELEMENTARY ____   HIGH SCHOOL _X_   COLLEGE ____   GRADUATE ____

PERSONAL PHYSICIAN _Dr. Fitness_    LOCATION _Activeville_

Reason for last doctor visit? _Check-up_ ____   Date of last physical exam _01_|_10_|_01_

Have you previously been tested for an exercise Program?  YES ___   NO _X_  YEAR (s) _—_ ____

LOCATION OF TEST ____ _—_ _____

Person to contact in case of an emergency _Bob_ _____  Phone # _123-4567_ (relationship) _husband_

### PLEASE CHECK YES or NO

| PAST HISTORY | | | FAMILY HISTORY | | | PRESENT SYMPTOMS | | |
|---|---|---|---|---|---|---|---|---|
| (Have you ever had?) | YES | NO | (Have any immediate family or grandparents had?) | YES | NO | (Have you recently had?) | YES | NO |
| High blood pressure ...... | ☐ | ☒ | Heart attacks ................. | ☐ | ☒ | Chest pain/discomfort .... | ☐ | ☒ |
| Any heart trouble .......... | ☐ | ☒ | High blood pressure ......... | ☐ | ☒ | Shortness of breath ....... | ☐ | ☒ |
| Disease of the arteries ... | ☐ | ☒ | High cholesterol .............. | ☐ | ☒ | Heart palpitations ......... | ☐ | ☒ |
| Varicose veins ............ | ☐ | ☒ | Stroke ......................... . | ☐ | ☒ | Skipped heart beats ...... | ☐ | ☒ |
| Lung disease .............. | ☐ | ☒ | Diabetes ........................ | ☐ | ☒ | Cough on exertion ........ | ☐ | ☒ |
| Asthma ...................... | ☐ | ☒ | Congenital heart defect ...... | ☐ | ☒ | Coughing of blood ........ | ☐ | ☒ |
| Kidney disease ............ | ☐ | ☒ | Heart operations .............. | ☐ | ☒ | Dizzy spells ................ | ☐ | ☒ |
| Hepatitis .................... | ☐ | ☒ | Early death .................... | ☐ | ☒ | Frequent headaches ...... | ☐ | ☒ |
| Diabetes .................... | ☐ | ☒ | Other family illness _____ | | | Frequent colds ............ | ☐ | ☒ |
| Heart murmur .............. | ☐ | ☒ | _osteo_ _____ | | | Back pain .................. | ☐ | ☒ |
| Arthritis .................... | ☐ | ☒ | _____ | | | Orthopedic problems ..... | ☐ | ☒ |

**(FOR STAFF)** _None < interview responses>_
_Race : caucasian_

**HOSPITALIZATIONS:** Please list recent hospitalizations (Women: do not list normal pregnancies)
Year          Location                  Reason
_2000_   _XYZ Hospital_   _Radical Hysterectomy (ERT)_

**Any other medical problems/concerns not already identified?** Yes ____ No _X_ (Please list below)

**Have you ever had your cholesterol measured?**  Yes **X** No ___ ; If yes, (value) **189** (Date) **10|01** Where? **XYZ**

**Are you taking any Prescription or Non-Prescription medications?** Yes **X** No ____ (include birth control pills)
Medication                              Reason for Taking                          For How Long?
___**ERT**_____     **Radical Hysterectomy**_____     **1 ½ yrs**_____

**Do you currently smoke?**  Yes ____  No **X**   If so, what? Cigarettes _____ Cigars _____ Pipe _____
How much per day:   < .5 pack ____     0.5 to 1 pack ____     1.5 to 2 packs ____     > 2 packs ____
**Have you ever quit smoking?** Yes ___ No **X** When? _____ How many years and how much did you smoke?

**Do you drink any alcoholic beverages?**  Yes **X** No ____ If Yes, how much in 1 week?
Beer _____ (cans)     Wine __**I**__ (glasses)     Hard liquor _____ (drinks)

**Do you drink any caffeinated beverages?**  Yes **X** No ____ If Yes, how much in 1 week?
Coffee **5** (cups)     Tea _____ (glasses)   Soft drinks _____ (cans)

<u>**ACTIVITY LEVEL EVALUATION**</u>
**What is your occupational activity level?**   sedentary **X** ;   light ____ ;   moderate ____ ;   Heavy _____
**Do you currently engage in vigorous physical activity on a regular basis?** Yes ____ No **X**
If so, what type? _____ How many days per week? _____
How much time per day? (check one)  < 15 min ____   15-30 min ____   30-45 min ____   > 60 min ____
Do you ever have an uncomfortable shortness of breath during exercise?   Yes _____ No **X**
Do you ever have chest discomfort during exercise?   Yes _____ No **X**  If so, does it go away with rest? ____
**Do you engage in any recreational or leisure-time physical activities on a regular basis?**  Yes ____   No **X**
If so, what activities? _____
On average:   How often? _____ times/week;   For how long? _____ time/session

**Are you currently following a weight reduction diet plan?** Yes ____ No **X**
If so, how long have you been dieting? _____ months  Is the plan prescribed by your doctor? Yes ____ No ____
**Have you used weight reduction diets in the past?** Yes **X** No ___ ; If yes, how often and what type?
___**Once, Weight Watchers for 3 months last year (01')**___

**Please indicate the reasons why you want to join the exercise program.**
To lose weight **X** Doctor's recommendation _____ For good health _____ Enjoyment _____
Release of tension _____ Improve physical appearance _____ Other **Energy / Youthful Feeling**
<u>**FOR STAFF USE:**</u>

**Blood Lipids : TC = 189 mg/dl    HDL = 49 mg/dl   Ratio = 3.86**
**TG = 196 mg/dl        FBG = 105 mg/dl**

Ms. Slimmer based on ACSM risk stratification before conducting an exercise evaluation on her.

Some 'important' pre-activity assessments on Ms. Slimmer include:##
  Resting heart rate (HR): 83 bpm
  Resting blood pressure (BP): 138/88 mmHg
  Blood profile:
    Total cholesterol: 223 mg/dL
    High density lipoprotein (HDL): 49 mg/dL
    Fasting blood glucose: 105 mg/dL

## Pre-Activity Screening (ACSM Risk Stratification Table)

In summary, Ms. Slimmer is a 45-year-old woman who is at low risk according to ACSM risk stratification (she has 1 ACSM risk factor— sedentary lifestyle) and, therefore, could perform most, if not all, health-related physical fitness assessments without any medical supervision. Of note: as a female under the age of 55 years, she is of lower risk of any complications during the exercise evaluations and a physician need not be present during those assessments.

ACSM Risk Stratification Table        Jane Slimmer

| | ACSM RF Thresholds | Comments | |
|---|---|---|---|
| — | Family History | No | (< 55/65 yo) |
| — | Cigarette Smoking | Never | |
| — | Hypertension | (138/88) | > 140/90 mmHg |
| — | Hypercholesterolemia | (189 mg/dl) | > 200 mg/dl |
| — | Impaired Fasting Glucose | (105 mg/dl) | < 110 mg/dl |
| — | Obesity | (26.2) | > 30 kg/m² |
| + | Sedentary Lifestyle | is not active for 30 minutes on most days | |
| — | HDL | (49) | < 60 mg/dl |
| 1 | (+) Risk Factors | | |
| 0 | Major Symptoms or Signs suggestive of C-P-M disease. | ⟨ denies all ⟩ | |
| Low | ACSM Risk Stratification | 1 = sedentary | |
| No | Need for Exercise Testing | not recommended | |
| No | GXT Physician Supervision | not recommended | |

## Body Composition Data (Anthropometry Data Form)

### Test Chosen: Body Mass Index (BMI)

Weight: 167 lbs (75.9 kg)
Height: 67 in (170.2 cm)
BMI: 26.2 kg·m⁻²

BMI calculation = $\dfrac{75.9}{1.702^2}$ = 26.19 kg·m⁻²

BMI interpretation: see Table 4-3 (OVERWEIGHT)

### Test Chosen: Waist-to-Hip Ratio (WHR)

Waist: 35 in (88.9 cm)
Hip: 37 in (94.0 cm)
WHR: 0.94

WHR calculation = $\dfrac{88.9}{94}$ = 0.946

WHR interpretation: see Table 4-4 (VERY HIGH)

### Test Chosen: 3-Site Skinfolds
Triceps: 17 mm

Abdominal: 25 mm

Suprailiac: 26 mm

SUM of 3 skinfolds = 68     SUM$^2$ = 4624

Percent body fat: 34.5%

Percent body fat calculation: (see Box 4-2 and Table 4-6 for formulas)

Body density (BD) = 1.089733 − 0.0009245 (68) + 0.0000025 (4624)

$\qquad$ − 0.0000979 (45 yo)

$\qquad$ = 1.089733 − 0.062866 + 0.01156 − 0.0044055

$\qquad$ = 1.0340215

Percent body fat $\quad = \dfrac{(5.01)}{1.0340215} - 4.5$

Percent body fat $\quad$ = 34.5%

Interpretation of percent body fat: see Table 4-5 (10–20$^{\text{th}}$ PERCENTILE)

---

### Anthropometry Data Form

Subject: __Jane Slimmer__  Date: __01/10/02__  Age: __45__ yrs

Gender: __F__  Technician: _____

Height: __170.2__ cm  __1.7__ meters Weight: __75.6__ kg

$\qquad$ __67__ in  $\qquad$ __167__ lb

Body Mass Index: __26.2__  Classification: _____

**Circumference Measurements (cm)**

| Site | 1 | 2 | 3 | Mean |
|---|---|---|---|---|
| Forearm | | | | |
| Arm | | | | |
| Abdomen | 88 | 89 | 89 | 89 |
| Waist | | | | |
| Hip | 94 | 95 | 94 | 94 |
| Thigh | | | | |
| Calf | | | | |

Waist to Hip ratio: __0.94__  Classification: _____

Waist Circumference: __89__  Classification: _____

**Skinfold Measurements (mm)**

| Site | 1 | 2 | 3 | Mean |
|---|---|---|---|---|
| Bicep | | | | |
| Tricep | 17 | 18 | 17 | 17 |
| Chest/Pectoral | | | | |
| Midaxillary | | | | |
| Subscapular | | | | |
| Abdominal | 24 | 26 | 25 | 25 |
| Suprailium | 26 | 26 | 26 | 26 |
| Thigh | | | | |
| Medial Calf | | | | |

% Body Fat __34.5__  Classification: _____

# Muscular Strength, Muscular Endurance, Flexibility Data Form

## Test Chosen: Sit and Reach Test

Results: 15 in
   Interpretation of flexibility: see Table 5-6 (~30th PERCENTILE)

## Test Chosen: Handgrip Test: 55 kg (combined left and right arms)

Interpretation of Muscular Strength: see Table 5-1 (BELOW AVERAGE)

## Test Chosen: Partial Curl-Ups

Results: 20 reps
   Interpretation of muscular endurance: see Table 5-4 (40th PERCENTILE)

---

### Muscular Strength, Muscular Endurance, Flexibility Data Form

Subject: __Jane Slimmer__   Date: __01|10|02__   Age: __45__ yrs
Gender: __F__   Technician: _____
Height: __170.2__ cm   Weight: __75.6__ kg
      __67__ in      __167__ lb

Muscular Strength: Hand-Grip   Dominant / Average / Combined

| Trial 1 (kg) | Trial 2 (kg) | Trial 3 (kg) | Best (kg) |
|---|---|---|---|
| 27 + 23 = 50 | 29 + 25 = 54 | 30 + 25 = 55 | 55 |

Classification: __Below Average__

Muscular Strength: 1 RM      Exercise: _____

| Trial 1 (kg) | Trial 2 (kg) | Trial 3 (kg) | Best (kg) |
|---|---|---|---|
|  |  |  |  |

Classification: _____

Muscular Strength: ISOKINETIC   Exercise: _____

| Trial 1 (kg) | Trial 2 (kg) | Trial 3 (kg) | Best (kg) |
|---|---|---|---|
|  |  |  |  |

Classification: _____

Muscular Endurance: Partial Curl-Up      Maximal

| Reps |
|---|
| 20 |

Classification: __40th Percentile__

Muscular Endurance: YMCA Bench Press      Maximal

| Reps |
|---|
|  |

Classification: _____

Muscular Endurance: Push-up      One Minute / Maximal

| Reps |
|---|
|  |

Classification: _____

Flexibility: Sit-n-Reach      Inches / Centimeters   Footline: _____

| Trial 1 (in / cm) | Trial 2 | Trial 3 | Best |
|---|---|---|---|
| 14" | 15" | 15" | 15" |

Classification: __~ 30th Percentile__

## Cardiorespiratory Fitness Data

*Test Chosen: Treadmill Graded Exercise Test Using Bruce Protocol*

Test time: 8:35 (8:35 = 8.58)

Other results: Ms. Slimmer had normal HR, BP, and ECG responses. She stopped the graded exercise test (GXT) as a result of fatigue. Her $HR_{max}$ was 187 bpm (her APMHR is predicted at 220 − 45 years old = 175 bpm (Figure 9-1).

$VO_{2max}$: 28.6 mL·kg$^{-1}$·min$^{-1}$

$VO_{2max}$ calculation: see estimate from Total Test Time Cubed Equation

$$VO_{2max} \text{ (mL·kg}^{-1}\text{·min}^{-1}) = 14.8 - 1.379 (8.58) + 0.451 (73.62) - 0.012 (631.63)$$
$$= 14.8 - 11.83 + 33.20 - 7.58$$
$$= 28.6 \text{ mL·kg}^{-1}\text{·min}^{-1}$$

---

**Maximal Graded Exercise Test Data Form**

Subject: Jane Slimmer       Age: 45 yr
Date: 10/25/02
Gender: F          Wt: 76 kg        Ht: 170 cm
                   167 lb           67 in
Protocol: Bruce      Mode: TM
Resting HR: 83 bpm          Resting BP: 138 / 88 mmHg

| Min | Workrate (mph/% grade) | HR (bpm) | BP (mmHg) | RPE | Comments |
|-----|------------------------|----------|-----------|-----|----------|
| 1 | 1.7 /10 | 98 | --- | | |
| 2 | | 109 | --- | | |
| 3 | | 115 | 152/90 | 9 | |
| 4 | 2.5 /12 | 132 | --- | | |
| 5 | | 149 | --- | | |
| 6 | | 161 | 168/92 | 14 | |
| 7 | 3.4 /14 | 185 | --- | | |
| 8 | | 187 | --- | (18) | (8:35) |
| 9 | | | | | |
| 10 | | | --- | | |
| 11 | | | --- | | |
| 12 | | | | | |
| 13 | | | --- | | |
| 14 | | | --- | | |
| 15 | | | | | |
| 16 | | | --- | | |
| 17 | | | --- | | |
| 18 | | | | | |

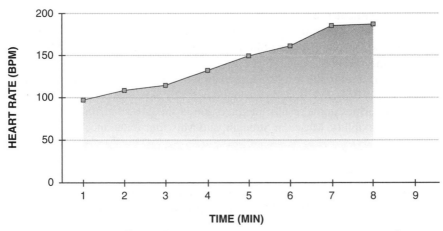

**FIGURE 9-1.** Heart rate for Jane Slimmer.

Interpretation of cardiorespiratory fitness: see Table 6-1 (~30th PERCENTILE)

Table 9-1 contains a summary of the test score interpretations for the health-related physical fitness tests.

As you gather all the health-related physical fitness test results together, you can decide on the best course of action for your client. Remember to consider the relative accuracies/practical applications of all the tests chosen when consulting with your client and when designing an exercise program to improve the test results. For example, muscular strength was assessed for Jane Slimmer using the handgrip test. There are other ways to assess muscular strength (see Chapter 5). Ms. Slimmer may achieve a different classification for muscular strength if a lower body assessment such as the leg extension test is used.

| TABLE 9-1 | HEALTH-RELATED PHYSICAL FITNESS SUMMARY FOR JANE SLIMMER | |
|---|---|---|
| **Test** | **Value** | **Classification** |
| ACSM Risk Stratification | 1 Risk Factor | LOW RISK |
| Body Mass Index | 26.2 kg.m$^{-2}$ | OVERWEIGHT |
| Waist-to-Hip Ratio | 0.946 | VERY HIGH |
| Percent Body Fat | 34.5% | 10–20th PERCENTILE |
| Flexibility (Sit and Reach) | 15″ | 30th PERCENTILE |
| Muscular Strength (Hand Grip) | 55 kg | BELOW AVERAGE |
| Muscular Endurance (Partial Curl-Ups) | 20 rep | 40th PERCENTILE |
| Cardiorespiratory Fitness (Bruce GXT − estimated $\dot{V}O_{2max}$) | 28.6 mL·kg$^{-1}$·min$^{-1}$ | 30th PERCENTILE |
| Cardiorespiratory Fitness (Bruce GXT − estimated $\dot{V}O_{2max}$) | 28.6 mL·kg$^{-1}$·min$^{-1}$ | 30th PERCENTILE |

## Questions

1. Does any one particular test or health-related physical fitness component stand out as any 'worse' or any 'better' than the others? In other words, what, if any, are the strengths and weaknesses for Jane Slimmer for the health-related physical fitness components measured/assessed?
2. Are there similarities in the results/interpretation of the body composition tests for Ms. Slimmer for BMI, WHR, and percent body fat by skinfolds?
3. Are there similarities in the results/interpretation of the muscular fitness tests for Ms. Slimmer for Flexibility, Muscular Strength, and Muscular Endurance?

## CASE 2: JOHN QUICK

Mr. Quick presents with the following tests results as found on the health-related physical fitness forms. Calculate all his results and interpret the test results for the following:

- Health History Questionnaire
- ACSM Risk Stratification Table
- Anthropometry Data Form
  - Body Mass Index
  - WHR
  - Percent Body Fat by 3-Site Skinfolds
- Muscular Strength, Muscular Endurance, Flexibility Data Form
  - Sit and reach
  - Handgrip
  - Push-Up
- YMCA Submaximal Cycle Ergometer Test Data Form
  - NOTE: It may have been recommended to Mr. Quick to have a maximal exercise test by ACSM Guidelines. He was also given a submaximal exercise test. See Figure 9-2 for a graph of the HR response to the exercise test.

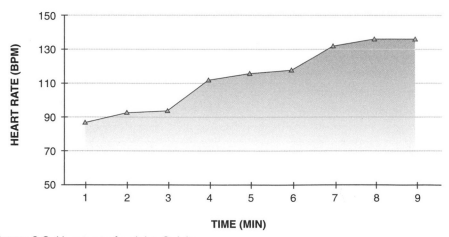

**Figure 9-2.** Heart rate for John Quick.

# Health-Related Physical Fitness Forms

## HEALTH HISTORY QUESTIONNAIRE

NAME John Quick    AGE 37    DATE 10|01|02 day/month/yr    DATE OF BIRTH 10|02|65 day/month/yr

ADDRESS 321 Oak Street Street    Inactiveville City    PA State    54321 Zip

TELEPHONE (home) 765-4321    (Business) 123-4567

OCCUPATION Salesman    PLACE OF EMPLOYMENT USA Products

MARITAL STATUS: (circle one)    SINGLE    (MARRIED)    DIVORCED    WIDOWED    SPOUSE: Ann

EDUCATION: (check highest level) ELEMENTARY ____    HIGH SCHOOL ____    COLLEGE X    GRADUATE ____

PERSONAL PHYSICIAN Dr. Sloth    LOCATION Inactiveville

Reason for last doctor visit? Check-up    Date of last physical exam 01|10|01

Have you previously been tested for an exercise Program? YES ___ NO X YEAR (s) _____

LOCATION OF TEST ___—___

Person to contact in case of an emergency Ann    Phone # 765-4321 (relationship) Wife

### PLEASE CHECK YES or NO

| PAST HISTORY | YES | NO |
|---|---|---|
| (Have you ever had?) | | |
| High blood pressure ...... | ☒ | ☐ |
| Any heart trouble ......... | ☐ | ☒ |
| Disease of the arteries ... | ☐ | ☒ |
| Varicose veins ............ | ☐ | ☒ |
| Lung disease ............. | ☐ | ☒ |
| Asthma ................... | ☒ | ☐ |
| Kidney disease ........... | ☐ | ☒ |
| Hepatitis ................ | ☐ | ☒ |
| Diabetes ................. | ☐ | ☒ |
| Heart murmur ............. | ☐ | ☒ |
| Arthritis ................ | ☐ | ☒ |

| FAMILY HISTORY | YES | NO |
|---|---|---|
| (Have any immediate family or grandparents had?) | | |
| Heart attacks ................. | ☒ | ☐ |
| High blood pressure ......... | ☒ | ☐ |
| High cholesterol .............. | ☒ | ☐ |
| Stroke .......................... | ☐ | ☒ |
| Diabetes ........................ | ☐ | ☒ |
| Congenital heart defect ...... | ☐ | ☒ |
| Heart operations .............. | ☐ | ☒ |
| Early death ..................... | ☐ | ☒ |
| Other family illness ___—___ | | |

| PRESENT SYMPTOMS | YES | NO |
|---|---|---|
| (Have you recently had?) | | |
| Chest pain/discomfort .... | ☐ | ☒ |
| Shortness of breath ....... | ☐ | ☒ |
| Heart palpitations .......... | ☐ | ☒ |
| Skipped heart beats ...... | ☐ | ☒ |
| Cough on exertion ........ | ☐ | ☒ |
| Coughing of blood ........ | ☐ | ☒ |
| Dizzy spells ................ | ☐ | ☒ |
| Frequent headaches ...... | ☐ | ☒ |
| Frequent colds ............ | ☐ | ☒ |
| Back pain ................... | ☐ | ☒ |
| Orthopedic problems ..... | ☐ | ☒ |

(FOR STAFF)

Family History - Father has heart disease (age 54); heart attack
Treated for High Blood Pressure
Had asthma as a child - no longer under treatment

**HOSPITALIZATIONS:** Please list recent hospitalizations (Women: do not list normal pregnancies)

Year    Location    Reason

None

_____

_____

*Any other medical problems/concerns not already identified?* Yes ____ No X (Please list below)

_____

_____

**Have you ever had your cholesterol measured?** Yes X No ___ ; If yes, (value) 178 (Date) 01/01 Where? hospital

---

**Are you taking any Prescription or Non-Prescription medications?** Yes ___ No ___ (include birth control pills)
Medication                              Reason for Taking                    For How Long?
Thiazide (diuretic)   for Blood Pressure          3 years

---

**Do you currently smoke?** Yes ___ No X   If so, what? Cigarettes ___ Cigars ___ Pipe ___

How much per day:   < .5 pack ___   0.5 to 1 pack ___   1.5 to 2 packs ___   > 2 packs ___

**Have you ever quit smoking?** Yes ___ No X   When? _____ How many years and how much did you smoke?

---

**Do you drink any alcoholic beverages?** Yes X No ___ If Yes, how much in 1 week?

Beer 3 (cans)   Wine _____ (glasses)   Hard liquor _____ (drinks)

---

**Do you drink any caffeinated beverages?** Yes X No ___ If Yes, how much in 1 week?

Coffee 14 (cups)   Tea _____ (glasses)   Soft drinks _____ (cans)

---

**ACTIVITY LEVEL EVALUATION**

**What is your occupational activity level?** sedentary X ; light ___ ; moderate ___ ; Heavy ___

**Do you currently engage in vigorous physical activity on a regular basis?** Yes ___ No X

If so, what type? _____ How many days per week? _____

How much time per day? (check one) < 15 min ___ 15-30 min ___ 30-45 min ___ > 60 min ___

Do you ever have an uncomfortable shortness of breath during exercise? Yes ___ No ___

Do you ever have chest discomfort during exercise? Yes ___ No ___ If so, does it go away with rest? ___

**Do you engage in any recreational or leisure-time physical activities on a regular basis?** Yes X No ___

If so, what activities? Golf (walk course)

On average: How often? 2 times/week;   For how long? ~120 min time/session

---

**Are you currently following a weight reduction diet plan?** Yes ___ No X

If so, how long have you been dieting? _____ months   Is the plan prescribed by your doctor? Yes ___ No ___

**Have you used weight reduction diets in the past?** Yes ___ No X ; If yes, how often and what type?

---

**Please indicate the reasons why you want to join the exercise program.**

To lose weight _____   Doctor's recommendation X   For good health X   Enjoyment _____

Release of tension _____   Improve physical appearance _____   Other _____

**FOR STAFF USE:**

ACSM Risk Stratification Table    John Quick

| | ACSM RF Thresholds | Comments |
|---|---|---|
| | Family History | (< 55/65 yo) |
| | Cigarette Smoking | |
| | Hypertension | > 140/90 mmHg |
| | Hypercholesterolemia | > 200 mg/dl |
| | Impaired Fasting Glucose | < 110 mg/dl |
| | Obesity | > 30 kg/m$^2$ |
| | Sedentary Lifestyle | is not active for 30 minutes on most days |
| | HDL | < 60 mg/dl |
| | (+) Risk Factors | |
| | Major Symptoms or Signs suggestive of C-P-M disease. | |
| | ACSM Risk Stratification | |
| | Need for Exercise Testing | |
| | GXT Physician Supervision | |

## Anthropometry Data Form

Subject: _John Quick_    Date: _10|1|02_   Age: _37_ yrs

Gender: _M_      Technician: _____

Height: _175_ cm    _1.75_ meters Weight: _72.7_ kg

       _69_ in                _160_ lb

Body Mass Index: _____      Classification: _____

**Circumference Measurements (cm)**

| Site | 1 | 2 | 3 | Mean |
|---|---|---|---|---|
| Forearm | | | | |
| Arm | | | | |
| Abdomen | 98 | 97 | 97 | 97 |
| Waist | 102 | 103 | 103 | 103 |
| Hip | | | | |
| Thigh | | | | |
| Calf | | | | |

Waist to Hip ratio: _____      Classification: _____

Waist Circumference: _____      Classification: _____

**Skinfold Measurements (mm)**

| Site | 1 | 2 | 3 | Mean |
|---|---|---|---|---|
| Bicep | | | | |
| Tricep | 16 | 17 | 16 | 16 |
| Chest/Pectoral | | | | |
| Midaxillary | | | | |
| Subscapular | 28 | 29 | 28 | 28 |
| Abdominal | | | | |
| Suprailium | | | | |
| Thigh | 23 | 24 | 23 | 23 |
| Medial Calf | | | | |

% Body Fat _____      Classification: _____

## Muscular Strength, Muscular Endurance, Flexibility Data Form

Subject: _John Quick_    Date: _10|1|02_    Age: _37_ yrs

Gender: _M_    Technician: _____

Height: _175_ cm    Weight: _72.7_ kg

_69_ in    _160_ lb

### Muscular Strength: Hand-Grip    Dominant / Average (Combined)

| Trial 1 (kg) | Trial 2 (kg) | Trial 3 (kg) | Best (kg) |
|---|---|---|---|
| 60 + 43 | 60 + 45 | 59 + 44 | 105 |

Classification: _____

### Muscular Strength: 1 RM    Exercise: _____

| Trial 1 (kg) | Trial 2 (kg) | Trial 3 (kg) | Best (kg) |
|---|---|---|---|
|  |  |  |  |

Classification: _____

### Muscular Strength: ISOKINETIC    Exercise: _____

| Trial 1 (kg) | Trial 2 (kg) | Trial 3 (kg) | Best (kg) |
|---|---|---|---|
|  |  |  |  |

Classification: _____

### Muscular Endurance: Partial Curl-Up    Maximal

| Reps |
|---|
|  |

Classification: _____

### Muscular Endurance: YMCA Bench Press    Maximal

| Reps |
|---|
|  |

Classification: _____

### Muscular Endurance: Push-up    One Minute / (Maximal)

| Reps |
|---|
| 24 |

Classification: _____

### Flexibility: Sit-n-Reach    (Inches) Centimeters    Footline: _____

| Trial 1 (in / cm) | Trial 2 | Trial 3 | Best |
|---|---|---|---|
| 15" | 16" | 16" | 16" |

Classification: _____

## YMCA Submaximal Cycle Ergometer Test Data Form

Subject: John Quick          Date: 10/01/02          Age: 37 yr

Gender: M          Wt: 160 lb 72.7 kg          Ht: 69 in 175 cm

Resting HR: 83 bpm          Resting BP: 132 / 78 mmHg * treated

Seat Height: 9          Predicted HR_max: 183 (220 − 37)

| Min | Stage | Work rate (kp·m·min$^{-1}$) | HR (bpm) | BP (mmHg) | RPE | Comments |
|-----|-------|------|------|------|------|------|
| 1 | I | 150 | 87 | | | |
| 2 | | | 93 | | | |
| 3 | | | 94 | 144/82 | 7 | — |
| | | | | | | |
| 4 | II | | 112 | | | |
| 5 | | 450 | 116 | 152/80 | 9 | — |
| 6 | | | 118 | | | |
| | | | | | | |
| 7 | III | | 132 | | | |
| 8 | | 600 | 136 | | | |
| 9 | | | 136 | 168/78 | 12 | — |
| | | | | | | |
| 10 | IV | | | | | |
| 11 | | | | | | |
| 12 | | | | | | |
| | | | | | | |

### Recovery

| Min | Active / Passive | HR (bpm) | BP (mmHg) | Comments |
|-----|------|------|------|------|
| 1 | Active | 122 | | |
| 2 | (150) | 116 | --- | |
| 3 | | 112 | 138/84 | |
| 4 | Passive | 98 | | |
| 5 | | 95 | | |
| 6 | | 92 | 128/78 | |

**In Summary: Essential Procedures: YMCA**

- ◆ Steady state Heart Rate (w/i ± 5 bpm) at workload
- ◆ Accurate Heart Rate measurement at workload
- ◆ Accurate workloads (check calibration and drift)
- ◆ 2 workloads that have Heart Rates between 110 - 150 bpm
- ◆ Accurate plotting of results

rev 10/00 GBD

## Calculating Test Results

It is recommended that you calculate and interpret all of Mr. Quick's test results and summarize the data in Table 9-2.

| TABLE 9-2  TEST INTERPRETATION FORM FOR JOHN QUICK | | |
| --- | --- | --- |
| **Test** | **Value** | **Classification** |
| ACSM Risk Stratification | | |
| Body Mass Index | | |
| Waist-to-Hip Ratio | | |
| Percent Body Fat | | |
| Flexibility | | |
| Muscular Strength | | |
| Muscular Endurance | | |
| Cardiorespiratory Fitness | | |

## Appendix A  Conversions

## LENGTH / HEIGHT

1 kilometer = 1,000 meters
1 kilometer = 0.62137 miles (1 mile = 1,609.35 meters)
1 meter = 100 centimeters = 1,000 millimeters
1 foot = 0.3048 meters (1 meter = 3.281 feet = 39.37 inches)
1 inch = 2.54 centimeters (0.394 inches = 1 cm)

## MASS OR WEIGHT

1 kilogram = 1,000 grams = 10 Newtons (N)
1 kilogram = 2.2 pounds (1 pound = 0.454 kilograms)
1 gram = 1,000 milligrams
1 pound = 453.592 grams
1 ounce = 28.3495 grams (1 gram = 0.035 ounces)

## VOLUME

1 liter = 1,000 milliliters
1 liter = 1.05 quarts (1 quart = 0.9464 liters)
1 milliliter = 1 cubic centimeter (cc or $cm^3$)
1 gallon = 3.785 liters

## WORK

1 Newton-meter = 1 Joule (J)
1 Newton-meter = 0.7375 foot-pounds (1 foot-pound = 1.36 Newton-meters)
1 kiloJoule (1000 J) = 0.234 kilocalories (kcal)
1 foot-pound = 0.1383 kilograms per meter (kgm) (1 kgm = 7.23 foot-pounds)

## VELOCITY

1 meter per second ($m \cdot sec^{-1}$) = 2.2372 miles per hour (mph)
1 mile per hour = 26.8 meters per minute ($m \cdot min^{-1}$) = 1.6093 kilometers per hour

## POWER

1 kilogram-meter per minute ($kg \cdot m^{-1} \cdot min^{-1}$) = 0.1635 Watts (W) (1 Watt = 6.1 $kg \cdot m^{-1} \cdot min^{-1}$)
1 $kg \cdot m^{-1} \cdot min^{-1}$ = 1 $kp \cdot m^{-1} \cdot min^{-1}$
1 Watt = 1 Joule per second ($J \cdot sec^{-1}$)
1 horsepower (hp) = 745.7 Watts

## TEMPERATURE

1 degree Celsius = 1 degree Kelvin = 1.8 degrees Fahrenheit (1 degree Fahrenheit = 0.56 degrees Celsius)

## METRIC ROOTS

deci = 1/10
centi = 1/100
milli = 1/1,000
kilo = 1,000

## CASE STUDY 1

A.A. is a 38-year-old sales representative, height 5'3", weight 185 lbs. His blood pressure is 150/80 mmHg, cholesterol 245 mg/dL, HDL cholesterol 56 mg/dL, triglycerides 80 mg/dL, and fasting blood glucose is 84 mg/dL. He volunteers his time as an emergency medical technician on an ambulance crew, which necessitates responding to calls at odd hours. He smokes recreationally and drinks at least two to three beers per day. He suffers chronic low back pain for the past 2 years. This low back pain occasionally necessitates him missing work. His father had a double bypass at age 62, and his sister has Type II diabetes. He initiated a weight-lifting program in his home 2 months ago and is now ready to continue his exercise program at your facility.

|   | ACSM RF Thresholds | Comments |
|---|---|---|
| − | Family History | Father @ 62 yo (< 55 yo) died of MI |
| + | Cigarette Smoking | Smokes recreationally |
| + | Hypertension | 150/80 mmHg > 140/90 mmHg |
| + | Hypercholesterolemia | 245 mg/dL > 200 mg/dL |
| − | Impaired Fasting Glucose | 84 mg/dL < 110 mg/dL |
| + | Obesity | BMI = 32.8 kg/m$^2$ > 30 kg/m$^2$ |
| + | Sedentary Lifestyle | Is not active for 30 minutes on most days |
|   | HDL | 56 mg/dL < 60 mg/dL |
| 5 | (+) Risk Factors |   |
|   | Major Symptoms or Signs Suggestive of CPM Disease | None present—asymptomatic |
|   | ACSM Risk Stratification | Moderate Risk |
|   | Need for Exercise Testing | Yes for vigorous exercise participation |
|   | GXT Physician Supervision | Yes for maximal GXT |

Notes: 38 yo or 'younger'

## CASE STUDY 2

B.B. is a 59-year-old insulin dependent diabetic for the past 4 years. Her health is well controlled through diet, exogenous insulin, and occasional walking. She is 5'2", 105 lbs, and very nervous. Her total cholesterol is 220 mg/dL, HDL 38 mg/dL, triglycerides 170 mm/dL, and fasting blood glucose is 120 mg/dL. She has been a secretary for more than 25 years. Leisure time activities include frequent trips with a social group at her church, and visiting her grandchildren. Her resting heart rate is 82 bpm and blood pressure 110/88 mmHg. Her father died at the age of 60 of a myocardial infarction, her mother is an active insulin dependent diabetic at the age of 81. She is here at the request of her physician, who recommended that she exercise regularly.

|   | ACSM RF Thresholds | Comments |
|---|---|---|
| − | Family History | Father died of MI @ 60 yo (< 55 yo) |
| − | Cigarette Smoking | No mention |
| − | Hypertension | 110/80 mmHg < 140/90 mmHg |
| + | Hypercholesterolemia | 220 mg/dL > 200 mg/dL |
| + | Impaired Fasting Glucose | 120 mg/dL < 110 mg/dL |
| + | Obesity | BMI = 32.8 kg/m$^2$ > 30 kg/m$^2$ |
| + | Sedentary Lifestyle | Occasional walking is not active for 30 minutes on most days |
|   | HDL | 38 mg/dL < 60 mg/dL |
| 4 | (+) Risk Factors | |
|   | Major Symptoms or Signs Suggestive of CPM Disease | No mention |
|   | ACSM Risk Stratification | High risk—IDDM |
|   | Need for Exercise Testing | Yes for moderate or vigorous exercise participation |
|   | GXT Physician Supervision | Yes for submaximal or maximal GXT |

Notes: 59 yo or 'older'

## CASE STUDY 3

C.C. is a 63-year-old male, who is a security guard. He is 5'7", 190 lbs, with a triglyceride level of 300 mg/dL, total cholesterol of 300 mg/dL, and blood pressure of 155/90 mmHg. He is a chronic television viewer who has never been "athletic" his entire life. He suffers from asthma, which is controlled by Ventolin. He avoids walking due to mild arthritis in his left knee. He smoked for 20 years before the asthma forced him to quit 2 years ago. He typically drinks two to three glasses of scotch a couple of evenings per week. Recently a graded exercise test was administered (Bruce Protocol) for complaints of chest pain. The test was terminated at stage two at a heart rate of 150 bpm due to volitional exhaustion. Additional testing revealed a hiatal hernia as the cause for the chest pain. He is at your facility because his physician suggests that he should exercise.

| ACSM RF Thresholds | Comments |
|---|---|
| Family History | (< 55/65 yo) |
| Cigarette Smoking | |
| Hypertension | > 140/90 mmHg |
| Hypercholesterolemia | > 200 mg/dL |
| Impaired Fasting Glucose | < 110 mg/dL |
| Obesity | > 30 kg/m² |
| Sedentary Lifestyle | Is not active for 30 minutes on most days |
| HDL | < 60 mg/dL |
| (+) Risk Factors | |
| Major Symptoms or Signs Suggestive of CPM Disease | |
| ACSM Risk Stratification | |
| Need for Exercise Testing | |
| GXT Physician Supervision | |

Notes: Chest pain is found to be from Hiatal Hernia, so CAD is 'ruled out.'

## CASE STUDY 4

D.D. is a 40-year-old administrative assistant with two small children, who suffers from chronic fatigue. She is 5′3″, 125 lbs, and is recently recovered from childbirth by cesarean section 5 months ago. She does not smoke and only ingests alcohol infrequently. Her resting pulse is 60 bpm with a resting blood pressure of 100/70 mmHg. She has engaged in exercise sporadically over the past 10 years, but complains of lightheadedness when she exerts herself. She also reports low back pain after performing Jane Fonda aerobics. Her cholesterol is 180 mg/dL and triglycerides are 100 mg/dL. Her mother was an insulin dependent diabetic at the age of 48 and her father suffers from osteoarthritis of the knee and low back. This client is interested in initiating an exercise program to increase her energy level.

| ACSM RF Thresholds | Comments |
|---|---|
| Family History | (<55/65 yo) |
| Cigarette Smoking | |
| Hypertension | > 140/90 mmHg |
| Hypercholesterolemia | > 200 mg/dL |
| Impaired Fasting Glucose | < 110 mg/dL |
| Obesity | > 30 kg/m$^2$ |
| Sedentary Lifestyle | Is not active for 30 minutes on most days |
| HDL | < 60 mg/dL |
| (+) Risk Factors | |
| Major Symptoms or Signs Suggestive of CPM Disease | |
| ACSM Risk Stratification | |
| Need for Exercise Testing | |
| GXT Physician Supervision | |

Notes:

## CASE STUDY 5

E.E. is a 30-year-old runner, height 5′10″, weight 165 lbs, who participates in road races bi-monthly. He works as a consultant with unusual hours and high stress. His resting heart rate is 40 bpm, and resting blood pressure 130/85 mmHg. Although he exercises regularly, his dietary intake consists of simple carbohydrates and at least a six beers daily. His total cholesterol is 245 mg/dL, triglycerides 450 mg/dL, and fasting blood glucose 100 mg/dL. Both of his parents were medicated for hypertension by age 50 and his father suffers from occasional gout. He suffers occasional shin splints and recurrent knee pain as a result of chondromalacia. The purpose of today's test is to monitor his health/fitness status.

| ACSM RF Thresholds | Comments |
|---|---|
| Family History | (< 55/65 yo) |
| Cigarette Smoking | |
| Hypertension | > 140/90 mmHg |
| Hypercholesterolemia | > 200 mg/dL |
| Impaired Fasting Glucose | < 110 mg/dL |
| Obesity | > 30 kg/m² |
| Sedentary Lifestyle | Is not active for 30 minutes on most days |
| HDL | < 60 mg/dL |
| (+) Risk Factors | |
| Major Symptoms or Signs Suggestive of CPM Disease | |
| ACSM Risk Stratification | |
| Need for Exercise Testing | |
| GXT Physician Supervision | |

Notes:

## CASE STUDY 6

F.F. is a 69-year-old male, who is retired from the New City Police Department. He is 5'9", 210 lbs, with a resting blood pressure of 140/80 mmHg. His family history reveals that his mother died of a myocardial infarction at age 70 and his father developed hypertension at age 70. At the present time he smokes approximately a pack of cigarettes a day and drinks beer and vodka daily. A recent blood test showed his cholesterol to be 260 mg/dL and high-density lipoprotein (HDL) to be 40 mg/dL. He does not complain of any orthopedic problems or chest pain. He had a myocardial infarction (MI) 6 years ago.

| ACSM RF Thresholds | Comments |
|---|---|
| Family History | (< 55/65 yo) |
| Cigarette Smoking | |
| Hypertension | > 140/90 mmHg |
| Hypercholesterolemia | > 200 mg/dL |
| Impaired Fasting Glucose | < 110 mg/dL |
| Obesity | > 30 kg/m² |
| Sedentary Lifestyle | Is not active for 30 minutes on most days |
| HDL | < 60 mg/dL |
| (+) Risk Factors | |
| Major Symptoms or Signs Suggestive of CPM Disease | |
| ACSM Risk Stratification | |
| Need for Exercise Testing | |
| GXT Physician Supervision | |

Notes: Myocardial infarction is a sign of coronary artery disease (CAD).

## CASE STUDY 7

G.G. is a 48-year-old male who is a sales representative for a large electronics firm. He travels quite a lot. He is 6'0", 190 lbs, with a resting blood pressure of 100/70 mmHg. Five years ago he has was diagnosed with Type II diabetes. He blames his 2½ packs per day smoking habit on the stress of his job. His family history reveals his brother had a MI at the age of 40. His cholesterol level is 250 mg/dL and HDL is 30 mg/dL. He complains of chest pain when he exerts himself.

His last exercise stress test was terminated due to shortness of breath and leg fatigue. He achieved 13 METS with a peak heart rate of 170 bpm and blood pressure of 160/90 mmHg.

| ACSM RF Thresholds | Comments |
|---|---|
| Family History | (< 55/65 yo) |
| Cigarette Smoking | |
| Hypertension | > 140/90 mmHg |
| Hypercholesterolemia | > 200 mg/dL |
| Impaired Fasting Glucose | < 110 mg/dL |
| Obesity | > 30 kg/m² |
| Sedentary Lifestyle | Is not active for 30 minutes on most days |
| HDL | < 60 mg/dL |
| (+) Risk Factors | |
| Major Symptoms or Signs Suggestive of CPM Disease | |
| ACSM Risk Stratification | |
| Need for Exercise Testing | |
| GXT Physician Supervision | |

Notes: Chest pain on exertion and shortness of breath (SOB) at end of maximal exercise test.

## CASE STUDY 8

H.H. is a 40-year-old male, height 5'7", weight 160 lbs. He is a grammar school teacher who is not particularly active because of pain in his knee that occurs as a result of an injury over 10 years ago. His blood pressure is 150/98 mmHg and total cholesterol is 210 mg/dL with HDL of 40 mg/dL. He does not smoke or drink and does not have any physical complaints other than his knee problem. Family history shows father developed coronary artery disease at age 60.

A previous Bruce Protocol test was administered. He achieved a peak heart rate of 183 bpm and blood pressure of 220/100 mmHg. The test was terminated due to claudication.

| ACSM RF Thresholds | Comments |
|---|---|
| Family History | (< 55/65 yo) |
| Cigarette Smoking | |
| Hypertension | > 140/90 mmHg |
| Hypercholesterolemia | > 200 mg/dL |
| Impaired Fasting Glucose | < 110 mg/dL |
| Obesity | > 30 kg/m$^2$ |
| Sedentary Lifestyle | Is not active for 30 minutes on most days |
| HDL | < 60 mg/dL |
| (+) Risk Factors | |
| Major Symptoms or Signs Suggestive of CPM Disease | |
| ACSM Risk Stratification | |
| Need for Exercise Testing | |
| GXT Physician Supervision | |

Notes: Claudication is leg pain related to CAD.

## CASE STUDY 9

J.J. is a 51-year-old bank executive who is 5'8" and weighs 182 lbs. He has been a heavy smoker all his life, but has admitted to quitting last week. He has Type II diabetes, blood pressure of 160/90 mmHg, and cholesterol is 246 mg/dL. He complains of chronic neck pain. He is also an occasional drinker. Family history reveals his mother had kidney failure at age 58.

He underwent a modified Bruce treadmill test, which was terminated due to shortness of breath at 4.2 mph and 16% grade. His peak blood pressure was 210/110 mmHg.

| ACSM RF Thresholds | Comments |
|---|---|
| Family History | (< 55/65 yo) |
| Cigarette Smoking | |
| Hypertension | > 140/90 mmHg |
| Hypercholesterolemia | > 200 mg/dL |
| Impaired Fasting Glucose | < 110 mg/dL |
| Obesity | > 30 kg/m² |
| Sedentary Lifestyle | Is not active for 30 minutes on most days |
| HDL | < 60 mg/dL |
| (+) Risk Factors | |
| Major Symptoms or Signs Suggestive of CPM Disease | |
| ACSM Risk Stratification | |
| Need for Exercise Testing | |
| GXT Physician Supervision | |

Notes: Shortness of breath (SOB) at intense exertion at end of maximal exercise test.

## CASE STUDY 10

K.K. is a 45-year-old white female, height 5'4", weight 120 lbs. She is president and owner of a cosmetic company. Her work demands many hours, including extensive travel. She is also divorced and the mother of 3. She smokes 2 to 3 packs of cigarettes per day and claims to drink 6 to 8 ounces of alcohol on most weekend nights. Her family history indicates her father suffered a fatal coronary embolism at age 60. The client claims she has little or no time to exercise, but wants to do something. Her resting blood pressure is 158/92 mmHg, her resting heart rate is 72 bpm, and total cholesterol of 215 mg/dL.

| ACSM RF Thresholds | Comments |
| --- | --- |
| Family History | (< 55/65 yo) |
| Cigarette Smoking | |
| Hypertension | > 140/90 mmHg |
| Hypercholesterolemia | > 200 mg/dL |
| Impaired Fasting Glucose | < 110 mg/dL |
| Obesity | > 30 kg/m$^2$ |
| Sedentary Lifestyle | Is not active for 30 minutes on most days |
| HDL | < 60 mg/dL |
| (+) Risk Factors | |
| Major Symptoms or Signs Suggestive of CPM Disease | |
| ACSM Risk Stratification | |
| Need for Exercise Testing | |
| GXT Physician Supervision | |

Notes:

**ANSWERS TO ACSM RISK STRATIFICATION CASES**

| ACSM RF Thresholds | 3 | 4 | 5 | 6 | 7 | 8 | 9 | 10 |
|---|---|---|---|---|---|---|---|---|
| Family History | – | – | – | – | + | – | – | – |
| Cigarette Smoking | – | – | – | + | + | – | + (last week) | + |
| Hypertension | + | – | – | – | – | + | + | + |
| Hypercholesterolemia | + | – | + | + | + | + | + | + |
| Impaired Fasting Glucose | – (n/a) | – (n/a) | – | – (n/a) | + NIDDM | – (n/a) | + | – |
| Obesity | – | – | – | + | – | – | – | – |
| Sedentary Lifestyle | + | + (?) | – | – | + | + | + | + |
| HDL | – (n/a) | – (n/a) | – (n/a) | – | – | – | – (n/a) | – (n/a) |
| (+) Risk Factors | 3 asthma pulmonary | 1 | 1 | 3 CAD | 5 NIDDM | 3 CAD | 5 NIDDM | 4 |
| Major Symptoms or Signs Suggestive of CPM Disease | Chest pain (?) | Lightheadedness | – | – | Chest pain, SOB | Claudication | SOB @ intense exertion (?) | – |
| ACSM Risk Stratification | HIGH | HIGH | LOW | HIGH | HIGH | HIGH | HIGH | MOD |
| Need for Exercise Testing (Vigorous) | YES | YES | NO | YES | YES | YES | YES | YES |
| GXT Physician Supervision (GXTmax) | YES | YES | NO | YES | YES | YES | YES | YES |

– (na) = not found

? = questionable (may need to use prudent judgment)

SOB = Shortness of breath

CAD = Coronary artery disease

NIDDM = Non-insulin dependent diabetes mellitus

MOD = Moderate risk

- Physical Activity Readiness Questionnaire (PAR-Q)
- Health History Questionnaire (HHQ)
- Sample Informed Consent
- ACSM Risk Stratification Table
- Anthropometry Data Form
- Muscular Strength, Muscular Endurance, Flexibility Data Form
- Maximum Physical Working Capacity Prediction
- Maximum Physical Working Capacity Prediction Example
- Submaximal Cycle Exercise Test Data Form
- Maximal Graded Exercise Test Data Form

Name: _____

Date: _____

# PAR-Q FORM

Many health benefits are associated with regular exercise, and the completion of PAR-Q is a sensible first step to take if you are planning to increase the amount of physical activity in your life.

For most people physical activity should not pose any problem or hazard. PAR-Q has been designed to identify the small number of adults for whom physical activity might be inappropriate or those who should have medical advice concerning the type of activity most suitable for them.

Common sense is your best guide in answering these few questions. Please read them carefully and check YES or NO opposite the question if it applies to you.

**YES** **NO**

☐ ☐ 1. Has your doctor ever said you have a heart condition <u>and</u> that you should only do physical activity recommended by a doctor?

☐ ☐ 2. Do you feel pain in your chest when you do physical activity?

☐ ☐ 3. In the past month, have you had chest pain when you were not doing physical activity?

☐ ☐ 4. Do you lose balance because of dizziness or do you ever lose consciousness?

☐ ☐ 5. Do you have a bone or joint problem that could be made worse by a change in your activity?

☐ ☐ 6. Is your doctor currently prescribing drugs (for example, water pills) for your blood pressure or heart condition?

☐ ☐ 7. Do you know of <u>any other reason</u> why you should not do physical activity?

---

If you answered **NO** honestly to <u>all</u> PAR-Q questions, you can be reasonably sure that you can:
1. Start a graduated exercise program
2. Take part in a fitness appraisal
However, if you have a minor illness (e.g.,cold) you should postpone activity.

---

If you answered **YES** to one or more PAR-Q questions, you should consult your physician if you have not done so recently before starting an exercise program and/or having a fitness appraisal.

---

**Physical Activity Readiness Questionnaire**

## HEALTH HISTORY QUESTIONNAIRE

NAME _____ AGE _____ DATE _____ DATE OF BIRTH _____
First        M.I.        Last                                    day / month / yr                              day / month / yr

ADDRESS _____
Street                                    City                          State        Zip

TELEPHONE (home) _____ (Business) _____

OCCUPATION _____ PLACE OF EMPLOYMENT _____

MARITAL STATUS: (circle one)    SINGLE    MARRIED    DIVORCED    WIDOWED    SPOUSE: _____

EDUCATION: (check highest level) ELEMENTARY _____ HIGH SCHOOL _____ COLLEGE _____ GRADUATE _____

PERSONAL PHYSICIAN _____ LOCATION _____

Reason for last doctor visit? _____ Date of last physical exam _____

Have you previously been tested for an exercise Program? YES ___ NO ___ YEAR (s) _____

LOCATION OF TEST _____

Person to contact in case of an emergency _____ Phone # _____ (relationship) _____

### PLEASE CHECK  YES  or  NO

| PAST HISTORY (Have you ever had?) | YES | NO | FAMILY HISTORY (Have any immediate family or grandparents had?) | YES | NO | PRESENT SYMPTOMS (Have you recently had?) | YES | NO |
|---|---|---|---|---|---|---|---|---|
| High blood pressure ...... | ☐ | ☐ | Heart attacks .................. | ☐ | ☐ | Chest pain/discomfort .... | ☐ | ☐ |
| Any heart trouble .......... | ☐ | ☐ | High blood pressure .......... | ☐ | ☐ | Shortness of breath ....... | ☐ | ☐ |
| Disease of the arteries ... | ☐ | ☐ | High cholesterol .............. | ☐ | ☐ | Heart palpitations .......... | ☐ | ☐ |
| Varicose veins ............. | ☐ | ☐ | Stroke ........................... . | ☐ | ☐ | Skipped heart beats ...... | ☐ | ☐ |
| Lung disease .............. | ☐ | ☐ | Diabetes ........................ | ☐ | ☐ | Cough on exertion ........ | ☐ | ☐ |
| Asthma ....................... | ☐ | ☐ | Congenital heart defect ...... | ☐ | ☐ | Coughing of blood ......... | ☐ | ☐ |
| Kidney disease ............. | ☐ | ☐ | Heart operations .............. | ☐ | ☐ | Dizzy spells ................ | ☐ | ☐ |
| Hepatitis .................... | ☐ | ☐ | Early death ..................... | ☐ | ☐ | Frequent headaches ...... | ☐ | ☐ |
| Diabetes .................... | ☐ | ☐ | Other family illness _____ | | | Frequent colds ............ | ☐ | ☐ |
| Heart murmur .............. | ☐ | ☐ | _____ | | | Back pain ................... | ☐ | ☐ |
| Arthritis .................... | ☐ | ☐ | _____ | | | Orthopedic problems ..... | ☐ | ☐ |

**(FOR STAFF)**

_____

_____

_____

**HOSPITALIZATIONS:** Please list recent hospitalizations (Women: do not list normal pregnancies)
Year                Location                              Reason

_____

_____

**Any other medical problems/concerns not already identified?** Yes ____ No ____ (Please list below)

_____

_____

*(continued)*

**Have you ever had your cholesterol measured?** Yes ___ No ___ ; If yes, (value) _____ (Date) _____ Where?

---

**Are you taking any Prescription or Non-Prescription medications?** Yes ____ No ____ (include birth control pills)
Medication                                        Reason for Taking                              For How Long?

---

**Do you currently smoke?** Yes ____ No _____ If so, what? Cigarettes _____ Cigars _____ Pipe _____

How much per day:  < .5 pack ____   0.5 to 1 pack ____   1.5 to 2 packs ____   > 2 packs _____

**Have you ever quit smoking?** Yes ___ No ___ When? _____ How many years and how much did you smoke?

---

**Do you drink any alcoholic beverages?** Yes _____ No _____ If Yes, how much in 1 week?

Beer _____ (cans)   Wine _____ (glasses)   Hard liquor _____ (drinks)

---

**Do you drink any caffeniated beverages?** Yes _____ No _____ If Yes, how much in 1 week?

Coffee _____ (cups)   Tea _____ (glasses)   Soft drinks _____ (cans)

---

**ACTIVITY LEVEL EVALUATION**

**What is your occupational activity level?**   sedentary ____ ;   light ____ ;   moderate ____ ;   Heavy _____

**Do you currently engage in vigorous physical activity on a regular basis?** Yes ____ No ____

If so, what type? _____ How many days per week? _____

How much time per day? (check one)  < 15 min ____   15-30 min ____   30-45 min ____   > 60 min ____

Do you ever have an uncomfortable shortness of breath during exercise?  Yes _____ No _____

Do you ever have chest discomfort during exercise? Yes _____ No _____ If so, does it go away with rest? ____

**Do you engage in any recreational or leisure-time physical activities on a regular basis?**   Yes ____   No ____

If so, what activities? _____

On average:   How often? _____ times/week;   For how long? _____ time/session

---

Are you currently following a weight reduction diet plan? Yes ____ No ____

If so, how long have you been dieting? _____ months   Is the plan prescribed by your doctor? Yes ____ No ____

**Have you used weight reduction diets in the past?** Yes ___ No ___ ; If yes, how often and what type?

---

Please indicate the reasons why you want to join the exercise program.

To lose weight _____ Doctor's recommendation _____ For good health _____ Enjoyment _____

Release of tension _____ Improve physical appearance _____ Other _____

**FOR STAFF USE:**

---

# Informed Consent

I, _____, have been told that I will perform a series of Health and Physical Fitness Assessment tests designed to aid in my understanding of my own health and physical fitness as well as enhance my understanding of these concepts. I understand that I have the freedom to withdraw from the testing at any time with no penalty. I also understand that I am free to ask any questions that may arise at any time and will have those questions answered to my satisfaction. Should any emergency arise during the testing, I understand that there is an emergency plan to follow. If I feel I have been injured from this assessment, I understand that I may contact _____ _____, with my concerns.

I have been told that I will perform a series of procedures and tests including a Health History Questionnaire, PAR-Q, , measurement of resting blood pressure, height, weight, body composition by _____, _____ for muscular strength, _____ for flexibility, _____ for muscular endurance, and a _____ for cardiorespiratory fitness.

There are few risks associated with these procedures and tests. The Health History Questionnaire, and PAR-Q involve no risks as they are pencil and paper tests. I understand that if I answer yes to any question on the PAR-Q test, I will not be tested on other procedures to ensure my safety. It has been explained to me that there is little risk with having my blood pressure, weight, and height measured. _____ . _____will be measured for body fat. While there is little risk associated with this, my right to privacy will be respected. The measurement of _____for flexibility, _____, and _____require some exertion on my part. However, there is little reported risks with these procedures. The _____ does involve near maximal exertion on my part and thus there is some risk associated with this test. The PAR-Q has been shown to screen out most potential complications for these types of tests. The most likely event to occur immediately after or within the first few hours after the test is local muscle soreness in the lower legs and knees. This should subside with time. I will report any and all signs and symptoms that I may have to _____ _____. I understand that all of my personal health and physical fitness data will be kept confidential. I am volunteering for these procedures and tests. I have read this form and understand both the form and the explanations given to me.

_____ .

Signature

_____

Date

_____

Witness

_____

Date

## ACSM Risk Stratification Table

|  | ACSM RF Thresholds | Comments |
|---|---|---|
|  | Family History | (< 55/65 yo) |
|  | Cigarette Smoking |  |
|  | Hypertension | > 140/90 mmHg |
|  | Hypercholesterolemia | > 200 mg/dL |
|  | Impaired Fasting Glucose | < 110 mg/dL |
|  | Obesity | > 30 kg/m² |
|  | Sedentary Lifestyle | Is not active for 30 minutes on most days |
|  | HDL | < 60 mg/dL |
|  | (+) Risk Factors |  |
|  | Major Symptoms or Signs Suggestive of CPM Disease |  |
|  | ACSM Risk Stratification |  |
|  | Need for Exercise Testing |  |
|  | GXT Physician Supervision |  |

## Anthropometry Data Form

Subject: _____ Date: _____ Age: _____

Gender: _____ Technician: _____

Height: _____ cm _____ meters Weight: _____ kg

_____ in _____ lb

Body Mass Index: _____ Classification: _____

| Circumference Measurements (cm) | | | | |
|---|---|---|---|---|
| **Site** | **1** | **2** | **3** | **Mean** |
| Forearm | | | | |
| Arm | | | | |
| Abdomen | | | | |
| Waist | | | | |
| Hip | | | | |
| Thigh | | | | |
| Calf | | | | |

Waist-to-Hip ratio: _____ Classification: _____
Waist Circumference: _____ Classification: _____

| Skinfold Measurements (mm) | | | | |
|---|---|---|---|---|
| **Site** | **1** | **2** | **3** | **Mean** |
| Bicep | | | | |
| Tricep | | | | |
| Chest/Pectoral | | | | |
| Midaxillary | | | | |
| Subscapular | | | | |
| Abdominal | | | | |
| Suprailium | | | | |
| Thigh | | | | |
| Medial Calf | | | | |

% Body Fat _____ Classification: _____

## Muscular Strength, Muscular Endurance, Flexibility Data Form

Subject: _____  Date: _____  Age: _____ yrs

Gender: _____  Technician: _____

Height: _____ cm  Weight: _____ kg

_____ in  _____ lb

Muscular Strength: Hand-Grip   Dominant / Average / Combined

| Trial 1 (kg) | Trial 2 (kg) | Trial 3 (kg) | Best (kg) |
|---|---|---|---|
| | | | |

Classification: _____

Muscular Strength: 1 RM   Exercise: _____

| Trial 1 (kg) | Trial 2 (kg) | Trial 3 (kg) | Best (kg) |
|---|---|---|---|
| | | | |

Classification: _____

Muscular Strength: ISOKINETIC   Exercise: _____

| Trial 1 (kg) | Trial 2 (kg) | Trial 3 (kg) | Best (kg) |
|---|---|---|---|
| | | | |

Classification: _____

Muscular Endurance: Partial Curl-Up   Maximal

| Reps |
|---|
| |

Classification: _____

Muscular Endurance: YMCA Bench Press   Maximal

| Reps |
|---|
| |

Classification: _____

Muscular Endurance: Push-up   One Minute / Maximal

| Reps |
|---|
| |

Classification: _____

Flexibility: Sit-n-Reach   Inches / Centimeters   Footline: _____

| Trial 1 (in / cm) | Trial 2 | Trial 3 | Best |
|---|---|---|---|
| | | | |

Classification: _____

NAME _____   AGE _____   WEIGHT _____ LB _____ KG   SEAT HEIGHT _____

|  | DATE | 1st WORKLOAD HR USED | 2nd WORKLOAD HR USED | MAX WORKLOAD | MAX O$_2$(L/min) | PREDICTED MAX HR | MAX O$_2$(mL/kg) |
|---|---|---|---|---|---|---|---|
| TEST 1 |  |  |  |  |  |  |  |
| TEST 2 |  |  |  |  |  |  |  |
| TEST 3 |  |  |  |  |  |  |  |

HR
200
190
180
170
160
150
140
130
120
110
100
90
HR

**DIRECTIONS**

1. Plot the HR of the 2 workloads versus the work (kgm/min).

2. Determine the subject's max HR line by subtracting subject's age from 220 and draw a line across the graph at this value.

3. Draw a line through both points and extend to the max HR line for age.

4. Drop a line from this point to the baseline and read the predicted max workload and O$_2$ uptake.

| WORKLOAD (kgm/min) | 150 | 300 | 450 | 600 | 750 | 900 | 1050 | 1200 | 1350 | 1500 | 1650 | 1800 | 1950 | 2100 |
|---|---|---|---|---|---|---|---|---|---|---|---|---|---|---|
| MAX O$_2$ UPTAKE (L/m) | 0.6 | 0.9 | 1.2 | 1.5 | 1.8 | 2.1 | 2.4 | 2.8 | 3.2 | 3.5 | 3.8 | 4.2 | 4.6 | 5.0 |
| KCAL USED (kcal/m) | 3.0 | 4.5 | 6.0 | 7.5 | 9.0 | 10.5 | 12.0 | 14.0 | 16.0 | 17.5 | 19.0 | 21.0 | 23.0 | 25.0 |
| APPROX MET LEVEL (for 132 lb) | 3.3 | 4.7 | 6.0 | 7.3 | 8.7 | 10.0 | 11.3 | 12.7 | 14.0 | 15.3 | 16.7 | 18.0 | 19.3 | 20.7 |
| APPROX MET LEVEL (for 176 lb) | 3.0 | 4.0 | 5.0 | 6.0 | 7.0 | 8.0 | 9.0 | 10.0 | 11.0 | 12.0 | 13.0 | 14.0 | 15.0 | 16.0 |

(continued)

NAME

AGE 33   WEIGHT 150 LB 68.2 KG   SEAT HEIGHT 12

DATE

PREDICTED MAX HR 187

|  | 1st WORKLOAD HR USED | 2nd WORKLOAD HR USED | MAX WORKLOAD | MAX O₂(L/min) | MAX O₂(mL/kg) |
|---|---|---|---|---|---|
| TEST 1 | 450- 128bpm | 600 142bpm |  | 2.45 | 35.9 |
| TEST 2 |  |  |  |  |  |
| TEST 3 |  |  |  |  |  |

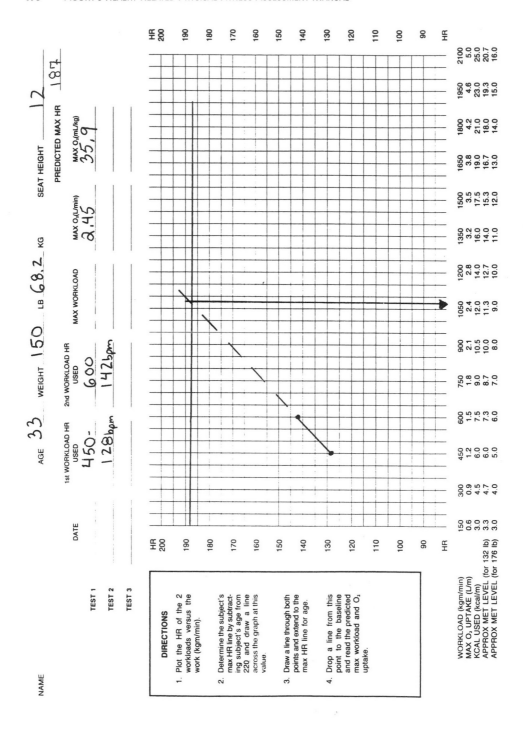

**DIRECTIONS**

1. Plot the HR of the 2 workloads versus the work (kgm/min).

2. Determine the subject's max HR line by subtracting subject's age from 220 and draw a line across the graph at this value.

3. Draw a line through both points and extend to the max HR line for age.

4. Drop a line from this point to the baseline and read the predicted max workload and O₂ uptake.

| WORKLOAD (kgm/min) | 150 | 300 | 450 | 600 | 750 | 900 | 1050 | 1200 | 1350 | 1500 | 1650 | 1800 | 1950 | 2100 |
|---|---|---|---|---|---|---|---|---|---|---|---|---|---|---|
| MAX O₂ UPTAKE (L/m) | 0.6 | 0.9 | 1.2 | 1.5 | 1.8 | 2.1 | 2.4 | 2.8 | 3.2 | 3.5 | 3.8 | 4.2 | 4.6 | 5.0 |
| KCAL USED (kcal/m) | 3.0 | 4.5 | 6.0 | 7.5 | 9.0 | 10.5 | 12.0 | 14.0 | 16.0 | 17.5 | 19.0 | 21.0 | 23.0 | 25.0 |
| APPROX MET LEVEL (for 132 lb) | 3.3 | 4.7 | 6.0 | 7.3 | 8.7 | 10.0 | 11.3 | 12.7 | 14.0 | 15.3 | 16.7 | 18.0 | 19.3 | 20.7 |
| APPROX MET LEVEL (for 176 lb) | 3.0 | 4.0 | 5.0 | 6.0 | 7.0 | 8.0 | 9.0 | 10.0 | 11.0 | 12.0 | 13.0 | 14.0 | 15.0 | 16.0 |

## Submaximal Cycle Exercise Test Data Form

Subject: _____          Age: ____ yr

Gender: _____          Wt: ____ kg          Ht: ____ cm

Protocol: _____          Cycle: _____

Resting HR: ____ bpm          Resting BP: ____ / ____ mmHg

| Min | Workrate (Watts) or $(kp \cdot m^{-1} \cdot min^{-1})$ | HR (bpm) | BP (mmHg) | RPE |
|-----|------|------|------|------|
| 0 | | | | |
| 1 | | | | |
| 2 | | | | |
| 3 | | | | |
| 4 | | | | |
| 5 | | | | |
| 6 | | | | |
| 7 | | | | |
| 8 | | | | |
| 9 | | | | |
| 10 | | | | |
| 11 | | | | |
| 12 | | | | |
| 13 | | | | |
| 14 | | | | |
| 15 | | | | |
| 16 | | | | |

**Recovery**

| Min | HR (bpm) | BP (mmHg) | Comments |
|-----|----------|-----------|----------|
| | | | |
| | | | |
| | | | |
| | | | |

# Maximal Graded Exercise Test Data Form

Subject: _____     Age:_____yr

Date: _____

Gender:_____     Wt: ___kg          Ht: ___cm

____lb               ___ in

Protocol: _____     Mode: _____

Resting HR:_____bpm          Resting BP: _____ / _____ mmHg

| Min | Workrate (mph/% grade) | HR (bpm) | BP (mmHg) | RPE | Comments |
|-----|------------------------|----------|-----------|-----|----------|
| 1   |                        |          | ---       |     |          |
| 2   |                        |          | ---       |     |          |
| 3   |                        |          |           |     |          |
| 4   |                        |          | ---       |     |          |
| 5   |                        |          | ---       |     |          |
| 6   |                        |          |           |     |          |
| 7   |                        |          | ---       |     |          |
| 8   |                        |          | ---       |     |          |
| 9   |                        |          |           |     |          |
| 10  |                        |          | ---       |     |          |
| 11  |                        |          | ---       |     |          |
| 12  |                        |          |           |     |          |
| 13  |                        |          | ---       |     |          |
| 14  |                        |          | ---       |     |          |
| 15  |                        |          |           |     |          |
| 16  |                        |          | ---       |     |          |
| 17  |                        |          | ---       |     |          |
| 18  |                        |          |           |     |          |

(*continued*)

## Recovery

| Min | HR (bpm) | BP (mmHg) | Comments |
|-----|----------|-----------|----------|
| 1 | | | |
| 2 | | | |
| 3 | | | |
| 4 | | | |
| 5 | | | |

# Index